Values and Ethics
for Care Practice

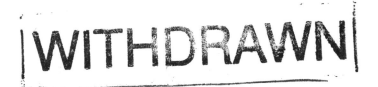

OTHER TITLES FROM LANTERN

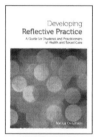

9781908625014

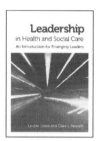

9781908625021

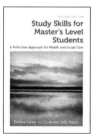

9781908625175

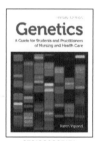

9781908625151

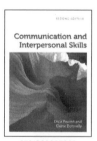

9781908625328

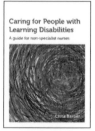

9781908625281

For more details see www.lanternpublishing.com

Values and Ethics for Care Practice

Sue Cuthbert & Jan Quallington
University of Worcester

Lantern

ISBN 9781908625304

First published 2017

This book is an updated and significantly expanded version of *Values for Care Practice* published by Reflect Press Ltd in 2008 (ISBN 9781906052058)

Lantern Publishing Limited, The Old Hayloft, Vantage Business Park, Bloxham Rd, Banbury, OX16 9UX, UK

www.lanternpublishing.com

www.cla.co.uk

British Library Cataloguing in Publication Data

A catalogue record for this book is available from the British Library.

The authors and publisher have made every attempt to ensure the content of this book is up to date and accurate. However, healthcare knowledge and information is changing all the time so the reader is advised to double-check any information in this text on drug usage, treatment procedures, the use of equipment, etc. to confirm that it complies with the latest safety recommendations, standards of practice and legislation, as well as local Trust policies and procedures. Students are advised to check with their tutor and/or mentor before carrying out any of the procedures in this textbook.

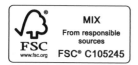

Typeset by Medlar Publishing Solutions Pvt Ltd, India

Cover design by Andrew Magee Design Ltd

Printed in the UK by The Complete Product Company Ltd

Distributed by NBN International, 10 Thornbury Rd, Plymouth, PL6 7PP, UK

CONTENTS

ABOUT THE AUTHORS

Dr Sue Cuthbert is the Head of Collaborative Programmes at the University of Worcester.

Sue qualified as an RGN and practised in care of the older adult and in women's health settings. Since moving into higher education in the 1990s, she has taught values and ethics in both nurse and midwifery education, as well as in applied health courses for undergraduate and postgraduate students. She now oversees the quality and delivery of a range of collaborative course developments with partner organisations, including Foundation Degrees in health and care.

She has an MA in Medical Ethics, where her research focused on reproductive choice, rights to healthcare, resource allocation and access to infertility treatment. She has since completed a Doctorate in Medical Ethics, also at Keele University. Her doctoral research examined the notion of choice in childbirth and competing models of autonomy in midwifery care, advocating for a pluralist view of values important to women's personal choices and decision-making, but where autonomy in midwifery practice is viewed through a social-relational lens.

Sue is also an informal family carer who has supported and cared for both her parents through the progressive effects of Alzheimer's and vascular dementia, and has therefore seen health and social care, both good and less satisfactory, from 'the other side'. This has further reinforced her conviction in the importance of practising values-based care and the centrality of respect, dignity and compassion for good holistic care.

Dr Jan Quallington is Head of the Institute of Health and Society at the University of Worcester.

Jan qualified as an RGN (Adult) and undertook specialist education in cardiothoracic nursing. Her clinical practice was in acute medicine, coronary care and intensive care. Since moving into education in a University setting Jan has studied for an MA in Medical Ethics and Law and has gained a Doctorate in Medical Ethics from Keele University. This focus on ethics has shaped the way that she thinks about practice.

Jan is passionate about educating and developing a workforce that will be effectively prepared to provide values-based, compassionate care. She believes that practitioners of the future must be confident to work collaboratively within a multiprofessional context, reflecting on and challenging with a view to leading, and enhancing practice.

Jan has undertaken a number of roles in higher education and has taught and learned from students across the health and social care spectrum. She currently leads a large multiprofessional team to deliver a wide range of health and social care education in partnership with health and social care providers and service users.

Jan has written on Ethical Reflection and on Leadership in health and social care.

PROLOGUE: ANNE'S STORY

Caring for other people is demanding and rewarding in equal measure. Good caring is not merely a practical intervention; it also requires a personal investment and quality of character that involves genuine concern and respect for others, but which gives the practitioner enormous personal satisfaction and sense of achievement when an intervention has gone well and made a difference to the patient.

Good care is built on positive values that enable therapeutic and human relationships with others to be forged. Care should rarely be something that is done *to* someone; rather it should be an activity undertaken in partnership with others – patients, families, carers and other practitioners and professionals. It would be arrogant to assume that any one individual has all the answers; consequently learning to work effectively in different kinds of partnerships will enable best care to prevail.

The relationship between care services, practitioners and patients, service users and their carers is a complex and interdependent one. Until relatively recently the care relationship was characterised by a model that positioned the 'professional expert' in a role that legitimised them as the decision-maker, selector and provider of the treatment and care. Priority was given to decisions that were perceived to be in the medical interest of the recipient who was, in turn, expected to be grateful and compliant in accepting and fulfilling the treatment expectations of that professional. Those who questioned this model or challenged decisions were at risk of being labelled difficult patients. In social care the model was slightly more embracing of the service users' perspective, but the service provider still acted as the final gate-keeper in determining which services the recipient would be able to access. Fortunately, more recently, it has been recognised that patients, service users and carers have much to contribute in achieving best outcomes and successful care episodes.

The involvement of patients and the public in health and social care has been a statutory requirement since the Health and Social Care Act of 2000 (HMSO, 2001). While service user and patient involvement is now widely acknowledged, and many would claim embedded, within services, its real potential is often not utilised. Engagement and involvement of patients and service users can be, at its worst, superficial and tokenistic, but where patients and service users work in partnership with professionals it can bring about practice that is person centred and effective for the patient, and indeed satisfying for the practitioner.

There are many ways of engaging people. Understanding how they experience services is fundamentally important in ensuring that the things that matter most to service users are incorporated into any care plan. One of the most commonly used ways of gauging patient experience of services is the 'Friends and Family Test'. This is a brief series of questions intended to ascertain the quality of an episode of care. While such a test might provide a blunt indication of a care experience as good or less than good, it does not provide the in-depth qualitative data about what and why something was good, and more importantly detail about what was not good. To really understand patient experience it is necessary to listen to people in their own words; to hear patient stories and to experience the world through their eyes. It is often the little things that seem unimportant to, or go unnoticed by practitioners that cause the most negative impact and annoyance to those in receipt of care.

People receiving care services are not generally predisposed to complain. As in all situations in life people expect to be treated with respect and consideration of their needs and most importantly, they want to be communicated with. This does not seem unreasonable and yet there are many stories of failure to achieve these few simple things. It is also true to say that if people are treated properly and communicated with, they will tolerate a greater degree of failure, lapses, and delays, far more readily than if they have been treated dismissively. Patients recognise that practitioners are normally doing their best, often in very busy and demanding environments. It would be disingenuous to say that people's expectations will always be met and that less than optimal situations and failures do not occur, because they do and they always will. However, if we can anticipate or recognise these situations and try to minimise their impact there is a much higher chance of the interaction with care services being positive, in spite of the circumstances. We cannot always get things right but how we try to, and how we deal with situations when we fail, will determine how the recipient experiences the situation. Really listening to and hearing others' perspectives and communicating effectively must always be the foundation of any interaction in care, whether you are busy or not. Treating people with due consideration and engaging in proper dialogue can prevent problems and frustrations later.

At the University of Worcester we believe service user and carer engagement is essential in helping future health professionals to understand the vital importance of partnership in care. We are committed to Service User and Carer engagement to inform and support all of our work and we are signatories to the National Involvement Partnership 4PI Standards. The service users and carers are a very committed team called IMPACT and their impact in supporting the education of future professionals is enormous. One of the members of this group, a carer and service user, Anne, volunteered to write and share some of her experiences of being in receipt of long-term care. We asked her to select a few examples from her interactions with care services. Anne has had very positive relationships and support from services over many years but she and her family have also been on the receiving end of endless, unnecessary frustrations. The things that she highlights as issues in the following piece are all avoidable, if practitioners take the time to listen to and respond appropriately, in partnership with those for whom we care.

ANNE'S STORY

Values in care practice: a service user's perspective

My son was born with microcephaly and a severe, profound learning disability. Although born at term, he was a low birth weight baby (4 lbs 15 oz) and spent several days in the special care baby unit. Although someone must have known about his condition at birth, when he was discharged from hospital we were given no indication that there was anything amiss. Nevertheless, it quickly became clear that things were not as should be expected; he did not meet any of the normal developmental milestones. He still does not have any speech, lacks mental capacity and requires a high level of help both day and night with washing, dressing, feeding, medication, mobility and all personal care needs. Over the years he has developed various other conditions including complex epilepsy and a severe back curvature. He is now 27; during the years that I have cared for him, over 50 different health and social care professionals have also been involved in his care. His care has, naturally, also involved numerous visits to doctors' surgeries, clinics, hospitals and other institutions, as well as very many home visits. It is frustrating how many times I have had to tell his story, each time we encounter a new practitioner, and yet how many different and inaccurate versions appear in his notes.

My son still lives at home with me, my husband and daughter, who are also very much involved with his care, and they too have contributed to these thoughts. I am myself a trained nurse, although I was unable to return to my career due to caring for my son.

What follows in this piece is not a series of criticisms and praises of health and care professionals but an attempt to relate my own experiences and align these to the values which should be evident in all health and social care practice.

There have been some real highlights, although often combined with less satisfactory instances. Take what happened when my son was first finally, formally diagnosed at six months. I had been concerned about him as soon as he was born but my concerns were always brushed aside. I had almost given up mentioning my worries as no one listened. However, when I took my son to have his second set of vaccinations, I did mention to the clinical medical officer that he had stopped smiling. Did this small remark ring alarm bells? Or was this doctor indeed 'actively listening' to me? What I do recall, to my immense relief, is that she actually did something constructive in response to my concerns. This leads me to reflect on the first fundamental value, that healthcare professionals must always actively listen to the patient and carers. Patients and carers hold many of the pieces of the puzzle, even if they do not know how to put them all together.

After examining my son, the doctor told me that she would not be giving him any more vaccinations at that time and that she was 'very worried' about him. She wrote a letter for me to take to the GP, 'straight away, don't wait'. Although I had worried that something was wrong I shall never forget the feeling of shock when this worry was finally acknowledged and shared; but then paradoxically came a highlight. My son's initial diagnosis was made on a Friday and even though it was the weekend, the GP contacted a Consultant Paediatrician who made it his responsibility to come round to our house on Saturday morning to see us and our son. Although he confirmed that there was global developmental delay, he then uttered the memorable words: 'There are lots of things we can do to help. Take each day as it comes and enjoy him!' (We have; and our son has a *joie de vivre* and a capacity to inspire which has enriched our lives and those of others.) This spontaneous but sincere remark really lifted our spirits, which were very low; later the consultant observed that when a person has learning disabilities 'their humanity shines through'. In a world often too obsessed with processes, referrals, paperwork and targets it is so important to show the service user and others that beyond all this lies a person with an inalienable dignity who matters, and this was a splendid example.

Looking back, I think that that this experience of first diagnosis epitomised a sense of teamwork and holistic care in which there was genuine compassion and a shared sense of purpose. We all had respect for one another's roles and in different ways we had all put ourselves out to do ordinary things in an extraordinary way.

A less satisfactory example of care occurred, also on a Friday. When our son was aged 19 he experienced a tonic–clonic epileptic seizure. For some time, the paediatrician had suspected that our son had developed epilepsy and although this suspicion had been documented, there was no conclusive diagnosis. However, our son had a seizure while out in the community. He came round from the seizure fairly quickly, but he looked pale and ill. We managed to get an emergency appointment at the GP surgery but were met by a skewed set of priorities. What apparently mattered was not concern about our son's condition but the doctor's concern for his own constraints: 'I've only got five minutes and I have other patients to see,' he said. We were dispatched home feeling dismissed and less important than other people. There was a vague mention of investigations at some stage but no information or any reassurance in spite of our obvious worry and distress.

How strange it is that a genuine health concern can be 'trivialised' or 'apparently disappear' particularly on a Friday, or during holiday periods, or when a young person moves from children's services to adult services, or moves between primary and secondary care services!

On reaching home, our son had a further serious tonic–clonic seizure and I rang for an ambulance. The paramedics were excellent: competent, practical, caring and showing the flexibility necessary when caring for someone with a learning disability and his carers. Yet once again in A & E we experienced a lack of empathy and understanding and regression to processes that actually hindered treatment. The staff in the A & E department were unable to adapt the care to meet his and our individual needs. I remember a nurse struggling to take our son's blood pressure, unnecessarily at that point, and causing him great distress while in the midst of another seizure; the doctor dismissing the paediatrician's diagnosis and other recent evidence rather than building on what was already known; the eventual appearance of anti-epileptic medication in tablet form, despite the fact that we had explained that our son could not swallow tablets. When we asked for the medication in liquid form, the explanation for failing to provide this was 'Oh, but the pharmacy is closed.'

What consideration was there for our son's individual needs in all this? Why so many barriers? Where was the common sense? How this was eventually resolved is too involved to explain here, but any feelings of trust and respect on our part were certainly casualties in that Friday surgery and subsequent A & E visit. Simply listening to us could have avoided such distress and a satisfactory outcome could have been reached much more quickly.

Each day for us is a learning curve: opportunities to say thank you when an appointment has worked well; the challenge of giving constructive advice when care hasn't gone well, or summoning up the courage to complain when all else fails. The capacity for us all to learn from one another is boundless, whether it is in formal teaching sessions or unwittingly in the course of face-to-face contact, treatment or in oral or written communication. The secret is that we must all be prepared to learn and to acknowledge that we do not have all the answers already: patients, carers and practitioners.

Communication is a double-edged sword that empowers and uplifts when done well, and demoralises and destroys when lacking in thought and compassion. We have endured bad moments when our son has thoughtlessly been described as 'defective', a 'naughty boy' (when having an epileptic seizure as an adult); or even been called by the wrong name altogether. Other highly insensitive remarks have been directed to me as a 24-hour, always-on-call, unpaid family carer: 'You don't do anything, do you?' I'm sure, however, that many remarks are thoughtless, rather than intentionally rude, and it does work both ways – any of us, including carers and service users, can irritate or infuriate, especially in moments of stress and frustration. How tempting it is to shoot the messenger when the system fails us; how difficult it can be sometimes to stay a 'professional professional' or a 'patient patient'! Long waits in outpatient departments spring to mind, with sharp words or assassinating looks from patients or staff, when an explanation and apology about waiting times is often all that is needed to defuse a difficult and often unavoidable situation. Not knowing is always more frustrating than a situation in which you have the information you need to make a plan; even if that plan is simply to go for a cup of coffee.

Take one more example: we took our son to an appointment at a hospital some 60 miles away. The appointment was for 9.30 am, even though we had said that our son would find such a long journey difficult, particularly at that hour (it took two hours in rush hour traffic). We explained that the examination and subsequent consultation would be more productive if the appointment could be at, say, 11 am. No, we were told, the consultant only saw new patients at 9.30 am.

In anticipation, we had made a dry run, without our son, to check car parking and the location of the clinic and the X-ray department, especially in view of the early start. We had also explained on numerous occasions that our son found X-rays difficult and asked whether we could please do some advance planning. However, we were told: 'It's only routine. We do these all the time'. It is ironic that professionals think that what is routine for them must also be routine for us.

What actually happened? We struggled to get there for the appointed hour and we found ourselves in a tiny airless cubicle with very bright lights, not suitable for anyone with epilepsy! The promised 'just another few minutes' turned into an hour, and soon we had to open the door so that we could breathe. Wretchedly, this compromised our son's dignity as the door led out onto a public area which afforded him no privacy. To add to this he was wearing an ill-fitting X-ray gown which had ties missing. In the end, as predicted, the routine X-ray could not be done; the type of equipment available was not suitable for someone with a severe learning disability. If we had been listened to at the start and messages passed on, then all this would have been avoided. Instead the experience and failure to X-ray our son not only compromised his dignity and delayed treatment, but also discriminated against him on account of his disability.

At all times, the dignity of each patient, service user and carer should be paramount, whatever the situation. In order to achieve this, any system needs to have an unashamed capacity to adapt in order to really care for individuals. It must have in-built flexibility that can accommodate different needs. It must learn to respect the experience of those who live with their condition, who are experts by virtue of their experience. Those working in care services need to keep reminding themselves: this person could be me!

To end, some little 'sight bites':
• Please listen to me
• Trust me and I'll trust you

- My time is important too!
- It's okay to say sorry – this works both ways
- I'm a person, not a process
- Short staffed should not mean short changed
- We're a team: all crew, no passengers.

Note from the authors

Anne has used just a few examples from the many interactions that she has had with care practitioners over the years. As she says, in her experience there is always going to be variability and things cannot always be perfect. However, reading the short list of 'sight bites' that she believes should accompany every care episode, we have to conclude that it is the small things that are often the most important and which make the most difference to those in receipt of care services. Ironically, these are the things that should easily be accommodated and which we would wish for if it were us receiving the care.

The basis of Anne's observations are simply a request that she, her family and her son are valued, listened to and treated with the dignity, compassion and respect owed to any person. Our reason for including Anne's experiences is to remind us that as practitioners we do not always know what frustrates others or how others experience the care we give, unless we ask them. This book aims to help practitioners to think about and reflect on value-based care and to ensure that the values discussed in this book really can be applied to the things that matter to patients and service users. We must never stop listening or assume that we always know best. At its best, care is a partnership of equals.

01

INTRODUCTION TO VALUES FOR CARE PRACTICE

LEARNING OUTCOMES:

In this chapter you will:

- Be introduced to the notion of values in care and distinguish between personal and professional values

- Establish the origin of values in care, including institutional and organisational influences, and explore those defined by professional bodies

- Recognise the significance of patient, service user and carer values

- Establish the importance of a plurality of values for health and social care and the need for practitioners to practise value-based reflection.

Values are an inescapable and integral feature of health and social care. Although not new, this claim was brought sharply back into focus through the findings of the Francis Inquiry which revealed unacceptable and appalling care, patients and families being treated with 'callous indifference', inadequate patient safety, and failures in leadership (Francis, 2013). Similarly, other reports of failures in hospitals and care homes have highlighted cases of poor, inhumane care (Care Quality Commission, 2014; Department of Health (DH), 2012b, 2013b; Keogh, 2013). All of these reports demonstrate incidents where values have been compromised in the provision and delivery of services and particularly in the standards of individual care. It appears that, at least for some, putting patients first had given way to other demands, in a culture that seemed to disregard the values of respect, compassion, dignity and person-centred care.

At the heart of what often troubles us in these narratives of mistreatment and inhumane care, is that our personal value position is challenged in some fundamental way. The actions of others in these scenarios are contrary to what we believe is the right way to behave and the right thing to do. We are shocked and appalled by the apparent disregard by others for the basic value of respect for individual people and humanity and the lack of any sense of compassion. There is an intuitive and emotional response and a need to make sense of others' and our own beliefs, values and behaviour. Care practice does not and should not occur in a moral vacuum and ethical behaviour is not reserved solely for the big issues, dilemmas and challenges in health and social care. Caring is based in the human relationship, and everyday activities and the simplest interactions or interventions have a moral component.

Lapses and failures in care are shocking and cannot ever be condoned, but neither must we make the mistake of suggesting that because some care fails, all care is failing. Most practitioners go to extraordinary lengths to defend and remain committed to their values (Calkin, 2011) and to ensure patients and service users receive excellent care (Jackson *et al.*, 2014; Middleton, 2013). What is clear is that the values held by practitioners are an essential component in determining and practising good care. It is also important to celebrate and promote good care whilst understanding how and why care can be compromised.

The Francis Inquiry (Francis, 2013) emphasised the importance of positive working cultures and the need for a workforce with the 'right values and attitudes' to provide high quality and safe care. There is an expectation of 'value-based recruitment and selection' of staff in health and social care; finding the person with the 'right' values to care (see the 'Cavendish Review' – DH, 2013d; Skills for Care, 2014; Willis Commission, 2012). Thus, in recent years, multiple claims have been made for the values that should guide the behaviours of health and care practitioners to ensure that all people using health and social care services are treated with respect and compassion and receive 'good care'.

Statements of values for health and care come from institutional, professional and organisational standpoints, both nationally and locally. A number of these have been significantly influenced by the 'patient or service user voice', either in a direct sense through consultation with individuals and user groups or through investigations and research into what people (and their families) want and expect when they receive care (Beresford, 2013; Burnell *et al.*, 2015; Cotterell *et al.*, 2010; Foot *et al.*, 2014; Lupton and Croft-White, 2013; National Voices, 2014; Tambuyzer and van Audenhove, 2015).

Examples of policy that incorporates value statements include 'The NHS Constitution' (DH, 2015a), the 'six Cs' (DH and NHS Commissioning Board, 2012c), 'Fundamental Standards' (DH, 2014c) and the Royal College of Nursing's Principles of Nursing Practice (RCN, 2011; see *Box 1.1*). Various professional organisations have codes and standards for practice which present collective value positions in defining the expectations of their professional group; for example, British Association of Social Workers (BASW), 2014; Nursing and Midwifery Council (NMC), 2015; Health and Care Professions Council (HCPC), 2016. This list is by no means exhaustive and although the values identified by each profession may be similar and interrelate, each organisation or body makes an independent claim. These values may also be defined at a high level and do not always identify their practical application in everyday decision-making and actions.

BOX — 1.1

The RCN principles of nursing practice

Developed in partnership with the Department of Health and the NMC, these describe what everyone, from nursing staff to patients, can expect from nursing. Nurses and nursing staff:

- treat everyone in their care with dignity and humanity – they understand their individual needs, show compassion and sensitivity, and provide care in a way that respects all people equally.

- take responsibility for the care they provide and answer for their own judgements and actions – they carry out these actions in a way that is agreed with their patients, and the families and carers of their patients, and in a way that meets the requirements of their professional bodies and the law.

- manage risk, are vigilant about risk, and help to keep everyone safe in the places they receive healthcare.

- provide and promote care that puts people at the centre, involves patients, service users, their families and their carers in decisions and helps them make informed choices about their treatment and care.

- are at the heart of the communication process: they assess, record and report on treatment and care, handle information sensitively and confidentially, deal with complaints effectively, and are conscientious in reporting the things they are concerned about.

- have up-to-date knowledge and skills, and use these with intelligence, insight and understanding in line with the needs of each individual in their care.

- work closely with their own team and with other professionals, making sure patients' care and treatment is co-ordinated, is of a high standard and has the best possible outcome.

- lead by example, develop themselves and other staff, and influence the way care is given in a manner that is open and responds to individual needs.

www.rcn.org.uk/professional-development/principles-of-nursing-practice

---

Deciding what is morally right to do in health and care, at policy and service levels and in practitioner–client relationships, has become an increasingly complex activity. This is influenced by the potential for competing personal and professional duties (for example, maintaining confidentiality and preventing harm), by advances in medicine such as genetic technology and by the ways in which limited health and social care resources are distributed. As Gallagher (2013, p.615) reminds us, '… organisational or political values, such as efficiency and effectiveness, may conflict directly with nursing values such as dignity, compassion and honesty'. Thus, practitioners have to find ways through this moral maze and the professional moral landscape to identify and prioritise the values for practice which they espouse and to determine the right ways to behave and act in the delivery of good care. Practitioners need to learn ways that challenge them to think critically and logically about their own and others' moral arguments and to derive morally defensible decisions that guide their practice. Although there may be more than one morally 'right' answer in many practice situations, what is important is that it is exposed to careful and critical ethical analysis and that actions can be morally justified. Authenticity in our decision-making comes when our espoused values are in alignment with those values that we exhibit in our actions, behaviours and attitudes.

In this book, readers will be encouraged to reflect on and critically analyse their personal value base and the core values underpinning health and care work. You will explore the origins of moral values in general and reflect on how these are articulated by organisations and in professional codes. You will consider how core values in health and social care give rise to principles that guide practice and reflect on cases where there are a plurality of relevant values for consideration and where values come into conflict. The text will use activities and case studies to enable the reader to reflect on the relevance of values in care practice and to apply theory in their practice.

This chapter introduces the notion of values in care and explores the distinction between personal and professional values. It considers the origin of values in care, including institutional and organisational influences, those defined by professional bodies and the significance of patient, service user and carer values. It concludes by emphasising the importance of a plurality of values for health and social care and the need for practitioners to practise value-based reflection.

INTRODUCING VALUES AND CARE

The very nature of health or social care work is that it is practical; it involves doing as well as understanding. You will need to *know that* something is the case, e.g. a fact of law or of anatomy and physiology, as well as *knowing how* to do something, e.g. a practical skill. The factual or knowledge base to perform the skills associated with health and care can be wide ranging, depending on your area of practice and level of expertise. For example, you may need to know how to perform urinalysis, how to safely move an immobile patient, how to listen effectively, how to apply a dressing to a wound, how to organise and run a group activity with service users, how to communicate with a person with hearing loss. You will learn the facts associated with '*knowing that*' and '*knowing how*' through teaching, inquiry and through practice.

Competence in practice also requires that you develop the relevant level of expertise, clinical and technical knowledge to assess an individual's needs and to provide safe, effective and quality care which is research- and evidence-based. Competence can be viewed as a holistic concept defined as 'the combination of skills, knowledge and attitudes, values and technical abilities that underpin safe and effective nursing practice and interventions' (NMC, 2010a, p.11 adaptation from Queensland Nursing Council 2009). While competence, efficiency and effectiveness are important components of care, these alone are insufficient to explain what it means to deliver good care; what matters is not just what you do but how you do it.

The verb 'to care' implies not merely a functional activity as, for example, the verb 'to run' may do, but also implies an activity that has a qualitative dimension. This dimension says something about the way in which caring is carried out. The verb 'to care' can be defined by using phrases such as: to be concerned about, to be watchful of, to have a liking for, to pay close attention to. Thus, caring is not a purely practical task that needs to be completed as efficiently as possible, but the implication is that the completion of the activity is undertaken with a particular attitude.

Caring requires a quality of character that involves genuine concern for the health, welfare and wellbeing of the individuals receiving care. In addition, while not universally true, many individuals receiving care may experience times of vulnerability, either by virtue of illness, age, disability, pain, or loss of confidence. Although we should be cautious in assuming that vulnerability demands protection and must avoid the creation of powerlessness or stigmatisation of individuals and groups in situations of vulnerability, patients, service users and their family carers may both expect and require support, advice and 'the care' of others. Thus, as care is essentially an interpersonal activity, caring about and for others requires not only knowledge and skills but a caring attitude that is value-based. It is the very nature of the care relationship and the ways in which we relate to others in our day-to-day practice that brings our value base into focus and demonstrates our respect for, and commitment to, others and their humanity. Knowledge and skills without values are directionless (Toon, 1999, p.58).

WHAT ARE VALUES?

Your personal beliefs and attitudes regarding how you should behave towards others, why you should act in a particular way, what is the right and wrong thing to do, are heavily influenced by your moral understanding, moral conscience and your values. Values are different from factual knowledge because they are harder to quantify, standardise or provide evidence of; however, their impact on the care relationship is fundamental. Put simply, values are particular kinds of beliefs that are concerned with the worth or value of an idea or behaviour and are important in guiding our actions, our judgements, our behaviour and our attitudes towards others. In this way, values play an essential role in articulating the standards for the delivery of care and the manner in which the practitioner interacts with others in the care relationship. The values explored in this book are those that dominate care in modern, western societies.

The concept of values may encompass a range of meanings and be understood in different ways and contexts, not all of which will be directly associated with morality. A value may describe an emotional disposition towards a person, object or idea, may be something we recognise as good or worthwhile, or reflect a personal belief or attitude about the truth, beauty or worth of a thought, object or behaviour (Pattison, 2004, pp.5–6). For example, when asked the value you attribute to a picture, you could respond by simply telling me how much it cost, you could talk about the reputation of the artist, you could say that it is beautiful and that you love it or you could tell me that it cost very little but it is priceless to you because of its sentimental value in reminding you of a special relationship.

Values may be used to describe the worth, importance or usefulness of something to someone. Seedhouse (2009, pp.48–9) identifies a number of categories of things we may attribute value to:
- Physical objects, e.g. our car, our house
- Aesthetic qualities, such as beauty, e.g. works of art, beautiful gardens
- Intangibles, e.g. friendships, creativity
- Principles or rules of behaviour, e.g. truth-telling, sanctity of life
- Ideologies, e.g. liberalism.

Pattison (2004, pp.3–5) outlines a number of synonyms used either in conjunction with, or instead of, the language of values:
- **Preferences, desires and choices** – from the economic domain, i.e. people value or confer worth on what they prefer, desire or choose (and are prepared to pay for).
- **Attitudes and beliefs** – from the psychological domain, i.e. what people are attitudinally or predisposed to, or believe in, is what they value and can be discerned by watching their behaviour, e.g. voting for a particular political party.
- **Social norms, assumptions, expectations, judgements and prejudices** – the sociological domain, i.e. what holds people together in groups so that society is coherent and individual behaviour is predictable; shared views of what is good or bad, desirable and undesirable.
- **Standards, visions and goals** – the domain of management and governance. Standards are norms of what is expected and required and define sufficient value, visions provide a set of ideal standards to which people can aspire, while goals are the intermediate specific value targets which must be reached.
- **Morals, principles and commitments** – the domain of morality and ethics. Morals are precepts or habits that aim to attain what is good and desirable, i.e. what is valued. Principles aim to ensure certain values are realised. Commitments are a form of consent to a set of values; the values you espouse and have committed

to follow, those you are morally obliged or compelled to observe and that guide your actions.

The definition of value is therefore multifaceted and complex. We will draw on all of the different expressions of values listed above. However, what is commonly meant when discussing values in health and social care (and is our main concern here) are the moral beliefs, principles or rules of personal conduct that guide our social interactions and human relationships. Humans are essentially social beings and individuals hold personal beliefs and values that are important to them and which influence their attitudes, actions and behaviours towards others. Our values in practice are also inextricably linked to the quality and acceptability of the care experience for those receiving care. Thus practitioners must not only identify with their own value base but should also respect and engage with the moral beliefs and position of others – the moral dimension of practice.

WHERE DO OUR BELIEFS AND VALUES COME FROM?

Much of our development of values and moral reasoning takes place during childhood and adolescence. These values may not be consciously selected or subjected to any scrutiny but inculcated from family and early socialisation or assimilated from cultural norms in education and play. Our development of moral knowledge is influenced by a number of factors including our parents and siblings, peer groups, culture, personality, education, religion and some form of ideology. Values are often subjective in nature, and can also be relative to the individual and their circumstances, culture, relationships and experiences. So, although our basic moral foundations of right and wrong, good and bad, what we ought or ought not to do are laid down in childhood, our values are not static and will inevitably be influenced by our experiences throughout life, including those values acquired from education, professional codes, organisations and working practices. Individuals may even reprioritise their values several times in the same day as they attempt to fit in with group norms or they will reprioritise their values at different stages of life or in response to various experiences. Yet there may also be some values that remain unchanged, that you are not willing to compromise and would take risks to defend.

Individuals are confronted with moral issues every day of their lives (not all to do with health or care). Requests for donations to charities, whether or not you recycle your rubbish, what you do when you are given too much change at the checkout, when your friend tells you about her affair with a colleague and asks you not to tell her husband. Many everyday circumstances and decisions have a moral component, so it should not be surprising that morality pervades your role and your decision-making as a practitioner in health or social care. Good, effective communication and interpersonal skills are essential throughout care practice; both in your work with patients, service users, clients, their families and carers and with other formal carers and professionals across a range of settings. What is also important is the moral dimension that comes into your decisions about how and what to communicate and a genuine caring attitude which will inevitably be influenced by your personal value position.

ACTIVITY 1.1

Reflection

Before you read the rest of this book it would be useful for you to reflect on your personal value and beliefs position.

Identify your core values; those beliefs that you hold that you would not be willing to compromise, e.g. that it is wrong to cause harm to another. Make a list.

Now order this list of personal values, placing the most important at the top.

Once you have 'rank ordered' your values, try to say why each is important to you. It may help to use the stem:

'I believe .... because ....'

For example, 'I believe it is wrong to intentionally harm someone else because I believe that life is precious and you should treat others how you would wish to be treated.'

You may think that the moral dimension is just a matter of intuition or common sense, not something that can or needs to be learned. While we all live by some personal value base, we do not always appreciate why we believe the things we do or we may be inconsistent in our values. There are often no clear or right answers, therefore reflection and further exploration are important elements of value-based care. The reality is that codes of practice identify broad guidelines or principles but cannot tell you how they should be applied in your everyday work or how to resolve issues where values conflict. Equally, you may have found it difficult to verbalise your core values and to provide justification for them in the activity above. Yet at some point you may be called to account regarding your moral judgements.

Great emphasis is placed on reflective practice in personal and professional development in health and social care. However, any critical reflection on your own and others' practice should start from the position of having identified and reflected on your own values. You will no doubt find that many of the things that trouble you (or deserve celebrating) in practice are those that challenge (or concur with) your personal value position. Identifying and prioritising your core values will help you to analyse issues in practice critically and to provide reasons or justifications for your value-based moral judgements.

Of course, we may not always live by the values we espouse (those we claim to believe and that define ourselves) and may instead defer to some other set of values; for example, those espoused by an organisation. At times, the practice of some individuals may fall below what are considered common standards of behaviour. This has been evident in a number of high-profile inquiries into healthcare organisations where staff have been found to have mistreated people or ignored their care needs, resulting in the abuse and neglect of patients and vulnerable people (DH, 2012b; Francis, 2013). As these cases demonstrated, the value position of leaders, managers and practitioners can be brought into question when care has gone so tragically wrong.

Moral values in health and social care can be observed on at least three different but interrelated dimensions; at the level of you as an individual (your moral integrity and being true to yourself), in your direct interactions with others (personal encounters and relationships; the value positions of others) and at a wider societal level, e.g. justice and fairness of groups or majorities. Although this book is chiefly aimed at exploring and reflecting on your personal values and how these influence your direct interactions with individuals in your care, the wider social morality inevitably influences your practice too. For example, how resources are distributed in health and social care and whether this is done fairly and justly will impact on your care decisions with individuals, even though you may feel that this is far removed from your realm of influence.

THE RELATIONSHIP BETWEEN PERSONAL AND PROFESSIONAL VALUES

Personal and professional values could be viewed as being distinct, in that your personal values may differ from those of another practitioner even though you belong to a specific care group and both observe the same code of practice. For example, your position on the moral status of the fetus and abortion may be very different from that of a colleague and yet you both work as maternity support workers with shared work values which may be influenced, although not bound by, *The Code: Professional standards of practice and behaviour for nurses and midwives* (NMC, 2015). Whatever you value in your personal life influences your moral conscience and behaviour and the judgements and decisions you make, which includes those made in your work. Thus, the boundaries between personal and professional values inevitably become blurred in their origin and influence.

You may also experience inconsistencies in your thinking, and reflecting on your beliefs may demonstrate that they cannot be adequately defended on logical, rational grounds. Equally, your personal values and principles may come into conflict with each other, giving rise to moral dilemmas in your own practice. For example, consider your beliefs about lying and truth-telling; do you always tell the truth? Or are there occasions when you evade telling the truth or consider 'a little white lie' as being permissible? Do you tell a friend that their new hairstyle looks ridiculous even if they are really pleased with it? When you are under-charged at the checkout by £10, do you point it out to the cashier? What about £1 ...or 1p?

Pattison (2004, pp.7–8) draws the distinction between 'normal' values and 'aspirational' values. What we are often referring to when we talk of values are the norms, rules, habits, expectations and assumptions that are at the heart of our social world and form the basis of social interaction and relationships. In this way, 'normal values' generally go unnoticed and require little or no justification or active commitment; they simply exist as part of the fabric of society. However, it is when these 'normal' values are challenged that passions rise and people become defensive, hurt and angry. Aspirational values are those that go beyond the norm; they are the beliefs and values that we would like to see integrated effectively in our own practice. This book provides the opportunity for you to consider in more depth those values that are fundamental to good care practice.

Groups of practitioners often hold or aspire to collective beliefs and common value positions concerning the ways they should behave and their duties and obligations to patients, service users and others. It may be that the kinds of people attracted to working in care roles come with some similarities in values and beliefs. There may also be specific external influences on both personal and professional values that come from defined institutional values and organisational culture, as well as those from a professional body and its code of conduct. In most countries, statements of professional values do not make direct reference to ideological, religious or political beliefs, although it is possible that specialist organisations might do so or in situations where culture and law are inextricably linked (Banks, 2012, p.8). However, it is important that we appreciate that not all value positions are good or lead to positive or beneficial outcomes for others. It is quite possible for individuals vehemently to defend their 'values' even though they may have disastrous consequences for others or exclude important concerns. Consider the example of extreme fundamentalism that believes it has the right to override the beliefs and values of others.

INSTITUTIONAL AND ORGANISATIONAL VALUES

Government bodies may set out collective institutional values which are intended to provide guidance on the core expectations for all workers within a given system or institution, with a view to influencing their attitudes and behaviours in practice. These institutional values may also be protected in law. The culture of organisations may also encompass a set of values and norms of the system. There may be explicit statements about the values and goals of the organisation and their commitments and contributions to society, the public, staff and those they serve.

In healthcare, the NHS Constitution for England (DH, 2015a) establishes the principles and values of the NHS, stating that patients should be at the heart of everything the NHS does, and espouses the values of respect, dignity and compassion (DH, 2015a, p.2). While the Constitution bestows legal obligations on healthcare practitioners and service providers to take account of its expectations in their decisions and actions, this does not 'guarantee' how or whether these values will translate into practice. What is legal need not necessarily cause someone to act morally; for example, consider how many people break the speed limit regardless of consideration for the safety of others or themselves.

As part of their response to the Francis Inquiry's recommendations, the UK government brought in legislation in 2014 which identifies fundamental standards and introduces a duty of candour for all health and social care providers from April 2015 (see *Box 1.2*). These 'fundamental standards' define the basic standards of safety and quality that should always be met with the intention of improving quality of care and ensuring that those responsible for poor care can be held to account, including criminal penalties without prior notice for a number of the standards. As regulatory standards, they provide an important protection for people, as well as a means for the Care Quality Commission (CQC) to take legal action to address poor care. The standards reflect the values enshrined within the NHS Constitution and extend to all health and social care provision.

BOX — 1.2

The Health and Social Care Act 2008 (Regulated Activities) Regulations 2014

Statutory Instrument 2014 No. 2936

The fundamental standards identified are:

- person-centred care – care and treatment must be appropriate and reflect service users' needs and preferences
- service users must be treated with dignity and respect
- consent – care and treatment of service users must only be provided with the consent of the relevant person
- care and treatment must be provided in a safe way
- service users must be safeguarded from abuse and improper treatment
- service users' nutritional and hydration needs must be met
- all premises and equipment used must be clean, secure, suitable and used properly
- complaints received must be investigated and necessary and proportionate action must be taken in response to any failure identified
- systems or processes must be established and operated effectively to ensure good governance
- sufficient numbers of suitably qualified, competent, skilled and experienced staff must be deployed
- fit and proper persons must be employed – persons employed must be of good character, have the necessary qualifications, skills and experience, and be able to perform the work for which they are employed
- registered persons must be open and transparent with service users about their care and treatment (the duty of candour).

It is regrettable that we need government-driven policy and legislation to remind us of some of the most fundamental and enduring values for health and care work. However, the Francis Inquiry (Francis, 2013) found in the majority of cases that significant harm could have been prevented if organisations had listened to the people in their care and their families and had practised according to some high standards underpinned by appropriate values. In the light of this and other independent inquiries into cases of abuse and neglect of vulnerable people, various Department of Health papers and reports claim to reinforce the fundamental values of healthcare. The White Paper

---

BOX 1.3

'The 6 Cs'

The six enduring values and behaviours that underpin *Compassion in Practice* (DH and NHSCB, 2012c) are defined as:

Care
Care is our core business and that of our organisations, and the care we deliver helps the individual person and improves the health of the whole community. Caring defines us and our work. People receiving care expect it to be right for them consistently throughout every stage of their life.

Compassion
Compassion is how care is given through relationships based on empathy, respect and dignity; it can also be described as intelligent kindness and is central to how people perceive their care.

Competence
Competence means all those in caring roles must have the ability to understand an individual's health and social needs and the expertise, clinical and technical knowledge to deliver effective care and treatments based on research and evidence.

Communication
Communication is central to successful caring relationships and to effective team working. Listening is as important as what we say and do and essential for 'no decision about me without me'. Communication is the key to a good workplace, with benefits for staff and patients alike.

Courage
Courage enables us to do the right thing for the people we care for, to speak up when we have concerns and to have the personal strength and vision to innovate and to embrace new ways of working.

Commitment
A commitment to our patients and populations is a cornerstone of what we do. We need to build on our commitment to improve the care and experience of our patients to take action to make this vision and strategy a reality for all and meet the health and social care challenges ahead.

Caring for our Future: reforming care and support (DH, 2012a) and the Department of Health paper *Compassion in Practice for Nurses, Midwives and Care Staff* (DH and NHSCB, 2012c) aimed to ensure that all health and social care services treat people with respect, dignity and compassion; the latter sets out a vision and shared purpose for nurses, midwives and care staff to deliver high quality, compassionate care, and to achieve excellent health and wellbeing outcomes. Regardless of developments and change in health and social care, 'what does not alter is the fundamental human need to be looked after with care, dignity, respect and compassion.' (DH and NHSCB, 2012c, p.5).

Through public engagement and consultation with health and care professionals, a set of values and behaviours, the '6 Cs' – care, compassion, competence, communication, courage and commitment – were identified and have been further enhanced by the publication of the Chief Nursing Officer's 'ten commitments' articulated in *Leading Change, Adding Value: a framework for nursing, midwifery and care staff* (NHS publications, 2016); see *Box 1.3*.

Not all of these might be considered to be 'moral values' in the philosophical sense. Nor do they define the only relevant values for healthcare practitioners. However, the interrelationship between the values of dignity, respect for persons and compassion and the ways in which these support other desirable attitudes and behaviours in care is clear (we explore these values in more detail in subsequent chapters). Courage and commitment may be seen as virtuous character traits for healthcare practitioners. Competence in practice, in the sense of technical, clinical and expert knowledge and skills, is clearly essential to the quality and effectiveness of care, as part of a duty of care and in the prevention of harms. All are underpinned by the need for good communication and interpersonal skills in all their forms to support the relationships essential to good care.

PROFESSIONAL BODIES AND CODES OF CONDUCT

Professions by their very nature often have their own cultures, their own bodies of knowledge and practice, and their own hierarchies and ways of working. For professional groups, the profession's collective value position may be defined by a particular professional body and described as a set of standards or in a code of conduct or practice.

For example, the NMC published their revised code of conduct, *The Code: Professional standards of practice and behaviour for nurses and midwives* (NMC, 2015) partly in response to the failings in care identified in the Francis Inquiry (Francis, 2013) but also to reflect modern healthcare practice and the ways in which patients' needs and the public's expectations of care have changed since the last Code of Conduct (NMC, 2008). It applies to student nurses and midwives as well as registered practitioners, researchers and educators, with a view to defining and ensuring consistent standards for conduct across the professional group. The Code is based around four key themes:

- Prioritise people;
- Practise effectively;
- Preserve safety;
- Promote professionalism and trust.

Each of these is divided into sub-themes which define the standards and what is required to meet them. Together these define the values of this professional group.

The Nursing and Midwifery Council (NMC) (NMC, 2010a) also identifies 'Professional Values' as one of the four domains of the 'Competency Framework' that defines the competencies every nursing student must acquire through their pre-registration nurse education programme in order to register as a practitioner with the NMC. The same standards are also published as *Standards for competence for registered nurses* (NMC, 2010b) and apply throughout a registered nurse's career.

Similarly, the Health and Care Professions Council (HCPC) is a regulator that sets out the standards of conduct, performance and ethics for all the professionals they register, including social workers in England.[1] Their *Standards of Proficiency* reflect both public expectations of professionals and the high standards that professionals expect of each other. The Social Work Reform Board (2012) developed the *Professional Capabilities Framework* (PCF) which defines the knowledge, skills and values that social workers need to practise effectively through every stage of their career (and how these should be developed during initial training). This is complemented by the British Association of Social Workers' *Code of Ethics for Social Work, Statement of Principles* (BASW, 2014).

ACTIVITY · 1.2

Comparing and contrasting professional codes

Locate a copy of the NMC *Code* (NMC, 2015) and the most recently published copy of the code of conduct or practice for two other distinct professional groups.

Identify the core themes in each.

Is there commonality in the language used? Are there distinctive features of each professional group? How are these expressed in the *Code*?

What are the similarities and differences in the values expressed in each of the codes?

The professional codes for nurses, midwives, allied health professionals and social workers identify the collective value base of each profession, and alleged cases of

---

[1]Arts therapists, biomedical scientists, chiropodists/podiatrists, clinical scientists, dietitians, hearing aid dispensers, occupational therapists, operating department practitioners, orthoptists, paramedics, physiotherapists, practitioner psychologists, prosthetists/orthotists, radiographers, social workers in England, speech and language therapists.

malpractice will be judged against the expectations of these Codes. And yet, if you look at several examples of Codes of Conduct or practice for professional groups, you will find that all members of the health and care professions share some common values and principles even if the practices arising from them are described in different ways. For example, social workers talk about anti-discriminatory practice, learning disability nurses about person-centred approaches, whereas adult nurses and midwives may emphasise respect for autonomy and the processes and practices that can help to achieve this, such as informed choice and woman-centred care. If you look beyond the differences in language you will see that all of these principles and practices are based in the values of respect for persons and humanity.

Although professional codes arise out of some sense of consensus morality and set the standards for the regulation of the profession concerned, they may be inflexible in their application to specific care situations and create dilemmas in practice where value statements are in conflict. Value conflict most frequently arises where a professional code demands that you act in the best interest, prioritise safety and promote wellbeing of the patient or service user while at the same time expecting that you respect their autonomy and facilitate personal choice. On the face of it, this seems unproblematic, but what if the patient in your care insists on using alternative or complementary therapy that there is no evidence to support or may be contraindicated with prescribed treatment? The Codes provide some broad statements of rules and duties to be observed but these alone may not assist in the adjudication of ethical decisions in everyday practice. We explore this further in relation to accountability (*Chapter 9*).

In view of the fact that values are so integral to the provision of care it is not just the 'typical' professional groups that have expressed values for practice. It has been recognised that care workers should be governed by a minimum set of values (Cavendish, 2013; Francis, 2013), and for this reason Skills for Care and Skills for Health (2013a) published a *Code of Conduct for Healthcare Support Workers and Adult Social Care Workers in England* and the *Core Competences for Healthcare Support Workers and Adult Social Care Workers in England* (Skills for Care and Skills for Health, 2013b). Although this Code is voluntary, it is seen as a sign of best practice and sets the standard of conduct and outlines the behaviour and attitudes expected of healthcare support workers and adult social care workers and their provision of safe, compassionate care and support. The Cavendish Review (2013, p.83) claims that society urgently needs a flexible, caring workforce with a common base of values and knowledge, proposing a 'Certificate of Fundamental Care' to make a positive statement about caring, and sees values as part of a 'golden thread' common to all workers in both health and social care (Cavendish, 2013, Recs 1, 3).

Patient, service user and carer values

Another key influence on how we practise is the value-base of those for whom we care. Practising patient or service user involvement and person-centred care should mean that practitioners are responsive to the individual's needs and values. Shared decision-making expects the practitioner to listen to and respond to the beliefs, values and preferences of those in their care (Elwyn and Charles, 2009). Establishing and taking into account the fact that patient or service user values and expectations about care might differ from your own is an essential component of care but can lead to dilemmas in care decisions. For example, one of the 'big issues' in society and in healthcare in the UK concerns requests for assisted dying, assisted suicide and voluntary euthanasia. Individuals who request assisted death may hold different understandings of what is in their best interests, leading to questions around the validity of their request and what it is to be autonomous and in control, and to make choices about the end of their lives.

Debates about the morality of some of the big issues in healthcare can expose differences in societal values and beliefs. However, often it is the small, seemingly insignificant things where differing value positions may impact most on the day-to-day care relationship, such as disapproving of a service user's style of dress, their refusal to wash or their choice of pastime, or using inappropriate humour. Listening to the voices of

---

BOX — 1.4

Caring for our Future: reforming care and support (DH, 2012a)

This was based on the views of people who use or who work in care and support across England. The consultation identified that a high quality care and support service must consist of the following linked core components:

- **Effectiveness** (good services make me feel better and more independent)
- **Positive experience** (good services treat me well)
- **Safety** (good services help to keep me safe)

A service cannot be judged to be good quality just because it is safe, if its effectiveness or people's experiences are ignored.

A high quality service means that people should say (p.37):

- I am supported to become as independent as possible.
- I am treated with compassion, dignity and respect.
- I am involved in decisions about my care.
- I am protected from avoidable harm, but also have my own freedom to take risks.
- I have a positive experience of care that meets my needs.
- I have a personalised service that lets me keep control over my own life.
- I feel that I am part of a community and participate actively in it.
- The services I use represent excellent value for money.

Extract from: DH (2012a, pp.36–37)

the patient, service user, their families and carers, identifying with their personal values and integrating these into the decision-making process is fundamental to our day-to-day value-based care practice. To do this, practitioners need to develop their own self-awareness and skills of interpersonal communication, have a broader knowledge and appreciation of service users' experiences and an understanding of moral values and ethics (Woodbridge and Fulford, 2004; Simons *et al.*, 2010).

ACTIVITY — **1.3**

> What moral values underpin the expectations of a high quality care and support service listed in *Box 1.4*?

As a health or care practitioner you are therefore faced with multiple claims for identifying the underpinning values essential to health and care. Gallagher (2013, p.615) has described this as a 'tsunami of values statements' and that we need to question the role and prioritisation of the many values that have been imposed on health and care professionals. Understanding the plurality of values at play in the healthcare encounter, and viewing health and care work as essentially an ethical enterprise forms the basis for ethical reasoning and the need to develop professional 'care' wisdom and judgement. Professional expertise develops from grappling with, reflecting on and finding solutions to the uncertainties, ambiguities and complexities in the 'swampy lowlands' of professional care practice where, '… messy, confusing problems defy technical solution' (Schön, 1987, p.3). This is not unique to the regulated 'professions' in health and care.

All health and care practitioners need to learn ways that challenge them to think critically and logically about their own and others' moral values and arguments in order to determine morally defensible care decisions and care practice.

CONCLUSION

There is no single definition of the term 'values' and it can be used in many ways. In a moral sense, values can be used to describe both the broader beliefs about the nature of a good society, such as a belief in the worth of human dignity, and more specific conduct-guiding principles that promote the belief, such as respect for an individual's autonomy (Banks, 2012, p.8). Our book will talk about values in both of these ways. In doing so, we aim to promote and help you to explore a range of significant values which we believe are fundamental to good care practice.

What we present is a plurality of relevant values for care work which allows for difference and diversity as well as the uniqueness of each individual care relationship. However, value-plurality means that decision-making is complex and methods must be employed to determine between competing values. At times there will not be one clear overriding value or principle to guide your actions; no singular 'morally right' answer to a practice dilemma. Decision-making will be both fact- and value-based.

An appreciation of ethics, ethical theory and ethical frameworks provides an essential addition to the toolkit for value-based critical reflection in and on practice for both the novice and experienced practitioner. *Chapter 2* provides an introduction to ethics and ethical theories which can be used in your deliberation of competing value positions and in making moral judgements and ethical decisions. The final chapter of the book (*Chapter 10*) promotes value-based reflection as a means to assist in this professional judgement and to arrive at morally sensitive care and ethically justified decisions and practice.

CHAPTER SUMMARY

Four key points to take away from Chapter 1:

- Caring is based in the human relationship and care practice does not and should not occur in a moral vacuum. Values are an inescapable and integral feature of health and social care, with both the simplest and most complex interactions and interventions having a moral component.
- Your personal beliefs and attitudes regarding how you should behave towards others, why you should act in a particular way, and what is the right and wrong thing to do, are heavily influenced by your moral understanding, moral conscience and values.
- Values are particular kinds of beliefs that are concerned with the worth or value of an idea or behaviour – the moral beliefs, principles or rules of personal conduct that guide our social interactions, our actions, our judgements, our behaviour and our attitudes towards others.
- Given the plurality of values relevant to the care relationship, decision-making can be complex and there may be more than one morally 'right' answer in any practice situation. Practitioners need to learn ways that challenge them to think critically and logically about their own and others' moral values and judgements and to derive morally defensible decisions that guide their practice. Value-based reflection is an essential part of the decision-making toolkit.

FURTHER READING

Banks, S. (2012) *Ethics and Values in Social Work*. 4th ed. Basingstoke: Palgrave Macmillan.

Duncan, P. (2010) *Values, Ethics and Health Care*. London: Sage Publications (particularly *Chapter 4 Ethical thinking: obligations and consequences*).

Seedhouse, D. (2009) *Ethics: the heart of health care*. 3rd ed. Chichester: John Wiley & Sons.

02

INTRODUCTION TO ETHICS FOR CARE PRACTICE

LEARNING OUTCOMES:

In this chapter you will:

- Establish what is meant by ethics and the distinction between morality and ethics, and clarify some key concepts relevant to ethical reasoning

- Identify the key features of different ethical theories commonly used in healthcare ethics

- Reflect on the relevance of ethics in supporting your moral judgements and decision-making in value-based health and care practice.

In *Chapter 1* we identified a range of influences on your development of personal and professional values and concluded that healthcare is essentially a moral enterprise in which a plurality of values are relevant to good care practice. However, recognising the importance of a number of different moral values means these can, at times, make competing demands on how you should behave and act. This requires you to determine whether the relevant values are equally weighted and mutually compatible or whether a decision needs to be made as to which value should take priority in guiding your actions in a given situation. The very nature of healthcare and the care relationship also brings with it the potential for moral problems and dilemmas (where the choice to be made involves conflict between different moral requirements or where alternative courses of action and outcomes are equally undesirable). Thus, all health and care practitioners need to learn ways that challenge them to think critically and logically about their own and others' moral values and arguments in order to determine morally defensible care decisions and responsible care practice.

This chapter clarifies what we mean by ethics, makes the distinction between morality and ethics and provides an insight into the relevance of ethics to value-based care.

It introduces and distinguishes between some key ethical concepts and theories often referred to in healthcare ethics. It aims to develop your understanding of ethics and ethical theories and their role in ethical reasoning, with a view to assisting your moral judgements and decision-making and supporting value-based critical reflection in practice for both the novice and experienced practitioner.

WHAT ARE MORALS AND ETHICS?

Both morality and ethical reasoning are at the heart of what it is to be a social being and to live in a society. Although it is common to use the language of 'morals' and 'ethics' interchangeably in healthcare literature, and the two are inevitably interconnected, they are distinct in meaning.

Morals and morality are concerned with the domain of personal values, beliefs, principles and rules of behaviour that influence and guide our social interactions and behaviours towards others. Our beliefs, values and morals are influenced by, and derived from, a number of different sources: our education, parents, religion, friends and social contacts, culture. Close inspection of these values and beliefs may reveal inconsistencies or conflicts; for example, we may have all learnt that it is wrong to lie yet questions of truth-telling (the 'little white lie') can arise in our everyday life as well as in the healthcare encounter. Thus, interrogation of our values and beliefs may demonstrate that they cannot always be adequately defended on logical, rational grounds.

In philosophical terms, ***ethics*** is about different ways of thinking about, understanding and examining how best to live a moral life (Beauchamp and Childress, 2013, p.1). It relates to the study and understanding of moral philosophy, morals and moral principles, the practical knowledge and skills in defining and applying the *principles* on which moral rules and values are based and the skills of *ethical decision-making*: applying moral theory and principles to practical situations and judgements of (morally) right or good actions.

It can help to understand ethics by considering what it is not:
- Ethics does not aim to describe how life is but how it should be. For example, sociological inquiry would be used to establish what women's attitudes are towards abortion, but ethics would consider whether abortion should be available, whether it is morally permissible and the rights and wrongs of abortion.
- Ethics is not the same as the law; morality may shape law, for example the cases of slavery and of homosexuality (although changes in morality take time to influence law, as is the case with law and abortion). That said, the law sometimes shapes morality, e.g. drink driving law, using seatbelts, mobile phone use and driving, reporting communicable diseases (using the law to influence behaviour in public health concerns).

- Ethics is not dependent upon religion or religious authority – you can be agnostic or atheist and have morals and behave morally. Although Judaeo-Christian traditions have played a dominant role in some cultures, they may no longer be universally accepted in a multicultural society. Similarly, some religious doctrines may not be in step with modern life, e.g. family structures, divorce, marriage of homosexual partners.
- Being ethical is not simply defined by observing a professional code – these form a statement of consensus morality and broad rules of a professional group but do not always determine an individual's morally right behaviour in specific circumstances.
- Ethical analysis is not the same as empirical scientific inquiry, science and technology – empirical inquiry sets out to establish facts and their validity and reliability, i.e. what is the case, whereas ethics is concerned with values and what ought to be. Scientific and technological development can also be relatively rapid in healthcare but what is scientifically possible may not necessarily be morally right or best (or at least requires careful consideration and strict parameters for its use), e.g. some advances in gene technology such as sex selection.
- Ethics is not about etiquette and custom – just because we have always done something that way does not mean it is the morally best or most desirable way.
- Ethical behaviour is not defined by policy – policies are driven by a number of factors including political ideology, political agendas, the media and pressure groups, and they do not necessarily reflect an ethical approach.

The term *ethic* may also be used as a noun, for example when referring to the collective belief- and value-system of any moral community, social or professional group; the ethos or '*spirit of a community*'. Professional codes of ethics generally define the professional ethic – the rules and standards of conduct of a professional group – and impose duties and responsibilities on the members of a specific profession that extend beyond those expected of the ordinary person. Thus the professional is also accountable for their actions and may be judged according to their professional code.

However, ethical behaviour requires more than the observance of the rules and standards within a professional code. Ethical decisions in healthcare are often made by practitioners in an individual encounter between themselves and the patient or service user. Thus, practitioners need to develop ways to regulate their own conduct and make decisions in their practice which are ethically defensible and would stand up to external scrutiny. Ethical awareness is an ongoing process requiring the exploration of our values and active deliberation and reflection on practice.

ETHICAL THEORIES AND PRINCIPLES

Ethical theories and principles provide a framework for questioning and reviewing our own and others' beliefs, values and moral behaviour. They can assist in decision-making by requiring the individual to think rigorously about a particular issue or aspect of care practice, evaluate different perspectives, articulate arguments and draw conclusions. Ethics does not necessarily give us one right answer to a moral problem or dispute but it can help to pinpoint where there may be conflict or disagreement in prioritising value positions, and elucidate the options or choices that are available.

Even though there may not be one 'right answer' to a given moral dilemma, there are systematic ways to examine our options, consider the evidence, clarify the underlying moral principles and the values at stake, and to act with forethought rather than impulsion or blind prejudice. 'As ethical professionals, our stringent moral responsibility is to *question* our taken-for-granted assumptions about the world, and not to presume they are always well-founded and unable to be challenged.' (Johnstone, 2009, p.105).

Completing *Activity 2.1* will help you to start to identify different ethical theoretical standpoints.

ACTIVITY **2.1**

What should Ryan do?

Ryan is a single parent of two young children. Money is tight and although he believes working to support his family is important, he has recently reduced his hours to look after his children. While paying for some food shopping at the self-service checkouts in one of a large chain of supermarkets, he realises that there is an extra £10 note in his change. In the moment, he thinks it's his lucky day; this will go towards his son's first pair of school shoes. There is no one around so he takes the change and leaves the store.

While driving home, he starts to reflect on what he has just done and thinks about what he would say if one of his children did something similar.

What kinds of arguments might he be thinking would defend his actions?

What kinds of concerns may be making him question his own judgement?

Initially, Ryan may have weighed up the consequences of taking the money. No one has seen what has happened and anyway they are a multi-million pound profit-making company; £10 is 'immaterial' as far as they are concerned. However, an extra £10 makes a significant difference to his personal finances and he has responsibilities to his children. For Ryan, the greater good for those immediately affected by his actions might seem to come from keeping the money. Plus, no one knows and he was not caught so no harm has come from it as far as his family is concerned.

He then wonders whether it was just a machine failure in giving him extra money or whether someone before him had not picked up their change. He feels less comfortable about this; it might have been someone more hard up than him. He resigns himself to the fact that he doesn't know this is the case and if it were, how could he identify the person? Surely they would have checked just as he had done (and if they realised later and were to be sufficiently demanding the company might well reimburse them in the spirit of good 'customer relations').

However, he then starts to think about what he would say if one of his children took money left on the table at home without asking him first. He would talk to them about deceit; that if they needed it, then they should ask otherwise it was a form of stealing; that if they took something from a shop, however small, that this was not only illegal but also morally wrong because it is taking something that does not belong to you; it is theft; that there are rules about how you should behave that determine whether actions are right or wrong and these include that you should not lie or steal, regardless of whether you might be caught. How would they feel if everyone behaved this way and stole from them? He realises that what he has just done is the same. Regardless of his initial motives and his belief that there were no immediate or obvious bad consequences, if everyone acted this way, we would not know who we could trust, and we may suffer harms as a result.

THE ROLE OF ETHICS

Moral values are an integral part of practice judgements. However, while clinical decisions may use scientific method to determine the best evidence-based practice, moral judgements are determined and justified in different ways. One approach to assist the critical evaluation of differing views, values and beliefs and to determine how to act morally is the application of ethical theories. Different ethical theories focus on different ways for judging what our obligations and duties should be and whether our decisions and actions are right or wrong, good or bad. Some make reference to rules and principles; some make value judgements of the potential outcomes; others focus on moral character and disposition.

Some philosophers have focused on producing a 'theory of morally right action' for ethical decision-making that can be applied universally in every similar situation and achieve consistent results when used by different people.

Consequentialism and deontology

Two such groups of ethical theory are **consequentialism** and **deontology**. 'Right' and 'good' are two important concepts in moral reasoning. In general, something is 'right' if it is morally obligatory whereas something is morally 'good' if it is worth having or doing (for wellbeing and happiness). These distinctions can be seen when comparing consequentialist and deontological theory.

Consequentialism involves identifying the consequences of our behaviour on others and includes utilitarianism (justifying actions on the basis of best consequences; the action that achieves the greatest good for the greatest number). On the other hand, **deontology** focuses on establishing the duties that we should follow (judgements that are based in moral duty or are rule based). Both of these may be evident in your deliberations of Ryan's actions. These theories are often cited in healthcare ethics and fall into a category of moral philosophy called **normative ethics**. Normative ethical theories aim to arrive at moral standards that regulate right and wrong conduct; to define the 'norms' of behaviour, how one should behave, what is ethically right or wrong action, what we should or should not do; our obligations and duties to others. A summary of key distinguishing features of these different theoretical approaches is provided in *Table 2.1*. If you want to know more about these ethical theories, further reading is identified at the end of this chapter (see also Duncan, 2010, Ch. 4).

Table 2.1 *Summary of key distinguishing features of different theoretical approaches to ethics*

Deontology (Kantian)	Utilitarian (a form of consequentialism)	Virtue ethics	Principle-based approach
Key proponent			
Immanuel Kant (1724–1804)	Jeremy Bentham (1748–1832) John Stuart Mill (1806–73)	Aristotle (4th century BC)	Beauchamp and Childress (1979, 2013)
Underlying assumptions			
Human beings are free, rational beings (i.e. autonomous); it is this moral agency that makes us intrinsically valuable Fundamental duty to respect all humans; human life has supreme value	Human beings are free individuals Living in society involves compromise of freedom	Virtue ethics focuses on inner character and motive and is therefore agent/person-based rather than action-based Do not disregard actions but have a distinctively virtue-ethics account of rightness/wrongness and good/bad actions Virtues are fundamental character traits needed to flourish or live well (duty and obligations are secondary)	Principles are derived from *common morality*, '...the set of norms that all morally serious persons share' (Beauchamp and Childress, 2001, p.3)
Ethical principles for determining moral action			
Takes **duty** to be the basis for morality (deon = duty)	**Consequentialism: predicted consequences or outcomes** of an action are used to judge whether the action is morally right or wrong	Concerned with the habits and knowledge of how to live a good life, i.e. **cultivating a virtuous character** and avoidance of moral incompetence	Principles not the same as rules as they allow room for more individual judgement

Deontology (Kantian)	Utilitarian (a form of consequentialism)	Virtue ethics	Principle-based approach
Concerned with moral duty and obligations; 'moral law' theory Rejects consequentialist claim; what is 'right' does not necessarily maximise happiness; prerogatives (or permissions) not to maximise the good Some actions are 'right' or 'wrong' by virtue of the act itself, irrespective of the consequences Fundamentally rule-based; **moral duties are categorical**, i.e. have the form of 'do x' rather than hypothetical, as in 'do x if you want y' Rules take the form of **prohibitions or constraints**, i.e. what I should NOT do, e.g. do not harm, do not lie May also include positive duties such as 'respect the autonomy of individuals' **Duties of special relationships** – duties arising from promises, contracts, friendships, parental relationships, professional role **Motive** for the action important; must intend what is morally required, e.g. refrain from stealing because morally wrong not because afraid will be caught Distinguish right action by asking 'Would I want all people to always act this way?'	Rightness and wrongness of actions judged according to the balance of their 'good' and 'bad' consequences An action is morally right if, and only if, it achieves the best available consequences **Utilitarianism:** the principle of **utility** (or 'usefulness') Choose the action that will achieve **'the greatest good for the greatest number'** Must choose the course of action which achieves the best, or least bad consequences, on balance, for all affected It is not about happiness for self but the happiness or interests of everyone affected by the action Utilitarians can justify allowing or even causing distress for some if the total amount of 'happiness' is maximised	**Developing the virtues is a necessary feature of living alongside others**; it is a social, political and moral feature of life, not just a personal one **Three key concepts in determining our moral character and competence as moral agents:** **Virtues** (and antithesis vice) **Practical or moral wisdom** *Eudaimonia* (human happiness or flourishing) An action is right if it is what a virtuous agent would characteristically do in the circumstances **A virtuous agent** is one who acts virtuously; someone who has, and exercises the virtues **A virtue is a character trait** a human being needs in order to flourish or live well For Aristotle **a good person is someone who lives virtuously**, i.e. who possesses and lives according to the virtues **Virtuous life is something that is practised and can be learned**; an internal state visible in our actions; we become virtuous through exercising the virtues consistently (not just habit but with intention and choice) Aristotle viewed **virtues as the mean between two extremes** (excess and deficiency) and strength of character involves finding balance between two extremes through reason (e.g. **virtue = compassion**; excess = 'bleeding heart'; deficiency = moral callousness)	Four principles are: **Autonomy** (the right to self-determination and respect for the decision-making capacities of autonomous persons) **Beneficence** ('doing good'; a group of principles requiring that we prevent harm, provide benefits and balance benefits against risks and costs) **Non-maleficence** (not causing harm to others) **Justice** (concerned with fairness; principles requiring appropriate distribution of benefits, risks and costs fairly) **Principles are not absolute and assume no prior ranking** Should be seen as binding principles to guide behaviour except where there is convincing evidence to suggest that they are inappropriate in a given instance When principles come into conflict, the prima facie or overriding principle takes precedence

(*continued*)

Deontology (Kantian)	Utilitarian (a form of consequentialism)	Virtue ethics	Principle-based approach
Never use people merely as a means to your own ends		The virtues identified should be attainable, i.e. the minimum set of characteristics that a person needs to possess in order to be regarded as virtuous For Aristotle, you cannot explain right and wrong simply in terms of rules BUT you can show how a virtuous person can be trusted to do the right thing in a variety of circumstances	
Examples of principles for practice supported by this theory			
Respect for autonomy and self-determination Person-centred care A duty of care Informed choice Informed consent Confidentiality	Promotion of welfare Maximising the public good, e.g. public health strategies such as smoking bans, vaccination Distributive justice, e.g. resource allocation according to the service or practice that maximises good	Compassionate care Courage – strength of character necessary to continue in the face of our fears. Courage combined with good judgement to take risks (e.g. whistleblowing, advocacy)	All of those identified opposite for deontology and utilitarianism

Principle-based approach

The **principle-based approach** (Beauchamp and Childress, 2013) has become one of the most commonly cited modern theories of bioethics in healthcare analysis. Principlism is an approach to ethics that arose out of the Belmont Report (1978) which concerned the protection of human subjects in relation to biomedical and behavioural research. The Belmont Report identified three principles (Respect for Persons, Beneficence and Justice) that were defined as general judgements that serve as the basic justification for the many ethical prescriptions and evaluations of human actions. These principles were adopted and expanded upon by Beauchamp and Childress firstly in 1979 (and most recently 2013) in their 'Principle-Based Approach to Biomedical Ethics'.

Beauchamp and Childress argue that the principles that have been selected arise from 'common morality', rather than having been arrived at by some theoretical method. On their account, a principle is 'an essential norm in a system of moral thought, forming the basis of moral reasoning' (Beauchamp, 2007, p.3). The principles identified in this theory are **Autonomy, Beneficence, Non-maleficence** and **Justice** (see *Box 2.1*).

BOX — 2.1

Beauchamp and Childress's Principles of Biomedical Ethics (2013, p.13)

Four 'clusters' of moral principles:

1. Respect for autonomy
   - respect for decision-making capacity of autonomous persons; respecting and supporting autonomous decisions

2. Beneficence
   - a group of norms pertaining to relieving, lessening, or preventing harm; providing benefits; balancing benefits against risks and costs
   - obligation to do good and to act in another's best interests

3. Non-maleficence
   - avoiding the causation of harm; obligation to not cause harms to others

4. Justice
   - Fairness; a group of norms for distributing benefits, risks and costs fairly.

These principles are not rules, which are specific in content and scope, and they are not absolute and assume no prior ranking. In this way, principles provide greater room for individual judgement. However, they should still be seen as binding principles to guide behaviour except where there is convincing evidence to suggest that they are inappropriate in a given instance. They may also be subject to further specification. When principles come into conflict, the prima facie or overriding principle takes precedence. More specific rules for healthcare ethics can be formulated by reference to these four principles. We will make reference to these principles in various ways throughout this book. For a succinct outline of the principle-based approach see Beauchamp (2007).

The principle-based approach could be said to offer a plurality of values to guide morally right action if each of the principles is taken to be equally weighted in value, as originally proposed by Beauchamp and Childress (2013). However, some references to this approach have raised respect for autonomy above all others, partly in an attempt to overcome the difficulties in adjudicating which principle should take precedence in guiding actions in any given situation (Gillon, 2003; Edwards, 2009). This primacy of autonomy has been reflected in healthcare practice through the last three decades with the assumption that if the patient (client, service user) is given the opportunity and supported to choose what is right or best for them, then the practitioner will have behaved ethically. However, this approach risks disregarding other values that are at least as important for consideration in good healthcare, such as protection from harm, trust, compassion.

Ethical theories that come from a liberal, rights-based tradition (such as deontology and utilitarianism), and to some extent the principle-based approach to biomedical ethics described above, give rise to what Fulford, Dickenson and Murray (2002, pp.1–2) call 'quasi-legal ethics'. This quasi-legal ethics has its focus in substantive ethical theory, ethical rules, regulation, the promotion of specific values, and in healthcare is often based in a medical–scientific 'fact-based' model of health. This is seen as mainly regulatory in purpose and gives attention to specific values, such as autonomy, rather than focusing on a diversity or plurality of values.

Although these kinds of theories may help us to arrive at normative 'morally right' answers, when dealing with humans at the heart of the care relationship these approaches seem insufficient in defining morally justifiable behaviour or in identifying what it is to be a good care practitioner. In the case of Ryan, you may have found yourself wanting or creating additional information about the kind of person Ryan might be and this may have influenced your decision about whether his approach was right or wrong. You may have wanted to know if he was a 'good' father; that although his actions on this occasion were essentially wrong, you may have identified other qualities that suggested he was generally of good character, 'virtuous' and commendable in his endeavours to support his young family. This would not condone stealing but might go some way to explain his weakness in this instance in his endeavours to be a good father.

Virtue ethics

Virtue ethics is another form of normative theory that provides an alternative approach to determining morally right behaviour without appeal to rules or consequences which are often counter to human nature and emotions. Instead, virtue ethics focuses on the moral agent in terms of your dispositions, intentions and motives and on the kind of person you are or want to become.

Virtue ethics starts from the questions, 'What sort of person should I be?' and 'What kind of life should I live?' Virtue theory can take account of human weakness (we do not always do what we ought to do) and the non-rational elements in the human character, like emotions and desires. The essential difference in virtue ethics is that the assumed norms are more concerned with our moral character and conscience and with certain traits (virtues) which are capable of being learned rather than in determining best consequences or in duty or obligation. Thus, virtue theory is chiefly concerned with moral character and with articulating the good habits that we should acquire. Virtue ethics is also a moral theory that can take account of emotions and an emotional response in ethical decision-making and action (Duncan, 2010, pp.89–90).

> 'The virtuous agent seeks and undertakes the good (virtuous) action … (and learns) … to become virtuous, to perform the good action, through following example, through observation of others and through reflection on my own experiences.'
>
> (Duncan, 2010, p.91).

Being of good character and pursuing a virtuous or 'good' life rather than one reliant on prescriptive rules therefore requires examination of both rational thought (cognition) and the affective domain of emotions and feelings. This seems attractive as an approach to healthcare ethics, particularly as we are concerned not only with what you should do or how you should behave morally speaking but also the kind of person you should be when involved in care practice and in your interactions with others in the care relationship.

Although we will talk a lot in this book about the values that influence your duties or obligations to others in your care, it is also important to consider what it is to be a 'good' practitioner. This can be expressed in terms of your moral character or virtues which incorporate a complex structure of habits, attitudes, beliefs, motives and emotions that encapsulate the positive values to which you aspire and impact on your personal judgements and actions. Beauchamp and Childress (2013, p.33) highlight some of the virtues often associated with health and care practitioners, derived both from social expectations and from standards and ideals internal to practitioner roles. These include the fundamental virtue of 'care' and five focal virtues which support and promote care and care-giving:

- Compassion
- Discernment
- Trustworthiness
- Integrity
- Conscientiousness.

Other relevant virtues include respectfulness, empathy, sincerity, truthfulness, benevolence, non-malevolence and faithfulness.

This list is by no means exhaustive but it starts to identify some of the standards and ideals of moral character important to health and care practice relationships. We might add wisdom (the need for sound judgement to inform practice) and courage (the courage to put your values into practice). Certainly, virtues such as courage, integrity, patience and respectfulness are central to good compassionate care. The antithesis of virtue is 'vice' and there may be some vices which are intolerable in the care relationship, such as callousness.

It is the practitioner's personal moral qualities that are of prime importance to service users, patients, clients and their families. However, the possession of virtues or good personal qualities by all practitioners cannot be prescribed because it is essential that these are deeply rooted in the person concerned and developed out of personal commitment rather than the requirement of an external authority. As Pattison (2004, p.5) suggests, being a virtuous (or good) practitioner is about more than simply following a set of rules (such as those that you find in Codes of Conduct or Practice). However, by adopting and conforming to certain values in the pursuit of particular visions or ends practitioners can become habitually virtuous such that the values, habits and attitudes become second nature and an essential part of the individual's character both in their everyday life and their practice.

Although some find virtue ethics problematic as an ethical theory for professional carers (see Holland, 2010), it seems to bring us one step closer to another important dimension in understanding what we should be concerned about in healthcare practice and educating health carers: that sense that providing 'good care' requires more than following abstract ethical rules; that there is something about the character of the caregiver, their relationship with the person receiving the care and the emotional impact of care that is important to their development of professional judgement and wisdom and is essential to becoming the good practitioner and caregiver.

CONCLUSION

This chapter has provided a brief introduction to the subject of ethics and its relevance to value-based care. Four different theoretical approaches to understanding normative ethics have been outlined and their distinguishing features identified. This has demonstrated that each theory places a distinct emphasis on the key ethical concepts of right and wrong, good and bad, duty and obligation and moral character (virtue and vice). However, all of these theories offer different perspectives on determining what is good for individuals and society, the norms of moral behaviour and what it means to lead the moral life. Understanding ethics and ethical theories and their role in ethical reasoning also provides a framework to explore moral problems and dilemmas in health and care and supports your deliberations, moral judgements and decision-making in practice, particularly where different values appear to conflict. In *Chapter 10* we promote 'values-led reflection' as an approach to analysing your own values base and examining the care you (and others) provide to your patients.

CHAPTER SUMMARY

Four key points to take away from Chapter 2:

- Ethics is the philosophical study of morality and considers how one ought to live and should act (morally speaking).
- Ethics is concerned with determining right and wrong conduct, good and bad actions and outcomes, duty and obligations and what we ought or ought not to do.
- Ethics (or moral philosophy) also seeks to systematically understand moral concepts, theories and principles and requires you to think rigorously about particular issues, problems or dilemmas, evaluate different perspectives and articulate your conclusions.
- Developing an understanding of ethics should assist your review of your own beliefs, values and moral behaviour and provides knowledge and skills that should deepen your reflections on practice.

FURTHER READING

Banks, S. (2012) *Ethics and Values in Social Work*. 4th ed. Basingstoke: Palgrave Macmillan.

Banks, S. and Gallagher, A. (2008) *Ethics in Professional Life. Virtues for health and social care*. Basingstoke: Palgrave Macmillan.

Beauchamp, T.L. (2007) The 'Four Principles' approach to health care ethics. *Chapter 1 in* Ashcroft, R.E., Dawson, A., Draper, H. and McMillan, J.R. (eds) (2007) *Principles of Health Care Ethics*. 2nd ed. London: John Wiley & Sons.

Beauchamp, T. and Childress, J. (2013) *Principles of Biomedical Ethics*. 7th ed. New York: Oxford University Press.

Duncan, P. (2010) *Values, Ethics and Health Care*. London: Sage Publications (particularly *Chapter 4*: Ethical thinking: obligations and consequences).

Seedhouse, D. (2009) *Ethics: The Heart of Health Care*. 3rd ed. Chichester: John Wiley & Sons.

Stanford Encyclopedia of Philosophy at http://plato.stanford.edu

This is an open access encyclopaedia maintained by Stanford University in the USA. It is aimed at those with a keen interest in philosophy, including applied philosophical ethics, and contains peer-reviewed and well-referenced papers written by recognised experts in the field. If you want a more in-depth insight into particular philosophical theories and concepts, then this is an accessible, well-recognised and refereed internet-based source. For example, search the site for entries on 'Care Ethics' (which takes you to a number of papers, including feminist ethics) and 'Virtue Ethics'.

Search for 'Autonomy' and you will find a paper entitled *Informed Consent* by Nir Eyal (2011) at http://plato.stanford.edu/entries/informed-consent/ (accessed 13 December 2016)

Search for 'Beneficence' and you will find *The Principle of Beneficence in Applied Ethics* by Tom Beauchamp (2013) at http://plato.stanford.edu/entries/principle-beneficence/ (accessed 13 December 2016)

03

COMPASSION AND CARE

LEARNING OUTCOMES:

In this chapter you will:

- Identify caring as a virtue and consider the moral attitude of caring behaviour

- Explore the patient, service user and carer perspective of experiencing good care

- Define and explore the meaning of the virtue of compassion

- Consider what it means to practise compassionate care

- Reflect on your and others' roles and responsibilities in providing compassionate care.

INTRODUCTION

As we saw in *Chapter 1*, a number of inquiries and reports have revealed a shocking lack of attention to the care needs of some of the most vulnerable members of our society. In particular, these reports identify examples of an appalling absence of the values of compassion, dignity and respect in caring for others. Thankfully, most care is not like that highlighted in these reports and very good care is frequently provided in spite of the many obstacles that surround it (CQC, 2011). Thus there is a question for practitioners, providers and educators to reflect on. How can we ensure that practitioners in every care episode consistently employ the values and associated attitudes and behaviours that should be at the heart of the care relationship?

One of the fundamental characteristics of 'good' care is that it requires not only the 'knowing-that' and 'knowing-how' to care but also demands a commitment to the caring process and a caring attitude. Benner (1984) views caring practice as that which involves both practical and attitudinal skills grounded in experiential knowledge, and pursued with the moral intent of bringing about good. The 'expert' practitioner practises in a way that combines the inner qualities of personal values and beliefs with cognitive and technical competencies.

In particular, the value of compassion has been identified as a necessary (if not sufficient) component of good care (DH, 2015a; DH, 2012a; DH, 2012c; Dewar, 2011, 2013; Francis, 2013; Youngson, 2008; Youngson, 2012). This chapter explores the value of care, what it means to be compassionate and how to practise and foster a culture of compassionate care.

CARING AS A VIRTUE

Caring is generally viewed as a virtue worth cultivating; people care, directly or indirectly, because they see this as valuable social behaviour. Society is a better place if we care for and about each other. It follows, therefore, that it should also be seen as a virtue in interpersonal professional work (Brykczyńska, 1997). Beauchamp and Childress (2013) view the virtue of care or caring (arising from an ethics of care) as being fundamental to the relationships, practices and actions of healthcare. They define caring as:

> '… care for, emotional commitment to, and willingness to act on behalf of persons with whom one has a significant relationship. *Caring for* is expressed in actions of "caregiving", "taking care of" and "due care".'
>
> (Beauchamp and Childress, 2013, p.35)

Similarly, Johnstone (2009, p.60), and Gastmans (1999) view 'good' (nursing) care as requiring more than mere competence. Gastmans *et al.* (1998, pp.45, 53) identify three fundamental components to the ethical view of nursing care as moral practice:
- the '*caring relationship*'
- caring behaviour as the '*integration of virtue and expert activity*'
- '*good care*' as the ultimate goal of nursing practice.

The essence of caring behaviour fundamental to good care is found in the integration of competence or expert activity with a 'virtuous attitude' of caring. Although this was identified in the context of nursing, it provides insights into what is important to the concept of 'good care' more generally.

> '…Caring as a moral attitude is perhaps less a matter of knowing how to act than of knowing how to be…'
>
> (Gastmans, 1999, p.218)

The level of practical skills and competence expected may vary according to your care role. However, there will still be defined skills and attitudes (caring behaviour) that should be present in the context of any particular caring relationship, with the intention or goal of providing 'good care' to the patient, client or service user. This goal of good care may include the promotion of the wellbeing of the person, not only in a physical sense but the psychological, relational, social, moral, and spiritual dimensions.

Begley (2010), in her reflections on what it is to 'be a good nurse', identifies certain virtues or attributes of the modern nurse that could equally be considered characteristic of any good 'professional' care practitioner (see *Figure 3.1*). These are categorised into three themes:

1. **Intellectual and practical wisdom** – the theoretical and practical wisdom of care practice which includes reasoning and judgement as well as knowledge, skills and competence
2. **Dispositional attributes** – the character or temperament of the carer
3. **Moral attributes** – the moral values underpinning care practice. (We would add respect for persons and dignity to Begley's 'list').

Many of these essential virtues such as trustworthiness, veracity, honesty and tolerance (see diagram in Begley, 2010, p.526) are not unique to care practice but define the morally 'good life' and 'living well' in Aristotelian terms. Being virtuous and of good moral character therefore brings something more to the notion of the good practitioner and good care than simply performing functions well and maintaining high standards in practice and governance (Begley, 2010, p.527).

VIRTUOUS CARING

Johnstone (2009, p.60) identifies two important consequences of 'virtuous caring' essential to 'good' moral (nursing) care practice:

1. Virtuous caring or 'right attitudes' are effective healing behaviours in the alleviation of human suffering and make a positive difference to a person's sense of wellbeing. These attitudes or behavioural orientations include compassion, empathy, concern, genuineness, warmth, trust, kindness, gentleness, nurturance, enablement, respect, mutuality, 'being there', attentive responsiveness, mindfulness, providing comfort, sense of safety and security.
2. Virtuous caring has a theoretical role for the moral motivation of care practitioners to act in beneficent ways. Thus rather than simply 'doing one's duty' as defined by duty-based theories (like deontology), in virtuous caring the motivation to act morally comes from moral sentiment, 'caring about' the person's wellbeing and alleviation of suffering. The 'caring practitioner' needs to be emotionally touched by what happens to the patient, both in a positive and a negative sense, and in a way that the cognitive and affective components of care inform one another.

Think about the notion of caring as a virtue in relation to *Activity 3.1*.

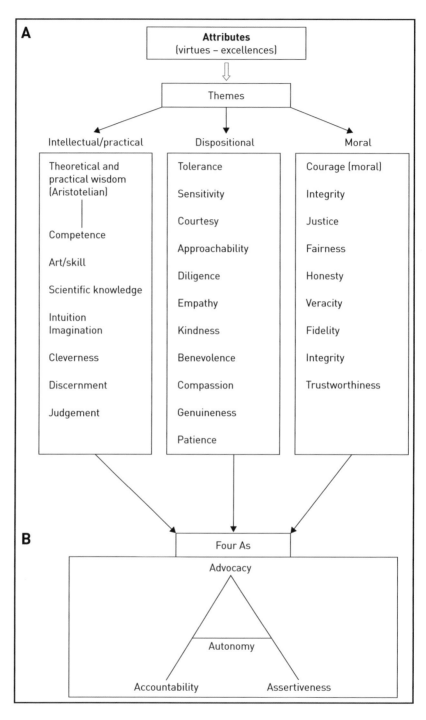

Figure 3.1 *Attributes of the modern nurse. Reproduced with permission from Begley (2010, p.526) On being a good nurse: reflections on the past and preparing for the future.* International Journal of Nursing Practice, *16: 525–532.*

ACTIVITY 3.1

Tender loving care (TLC)?

An elderly woman is admitted from A & E to an acute admissions unit following a fall. She is being monitored and receiving drug treatment for newly diagnosed heart failure that may have contributed to her falling. A relative visits and finds the woman upset because she has spilt her soup and tea down her nightdress and the bedding; the woman says it is her 'own fault' because she couldn't hold the cup whilst lying on her side but she is uncomfortable in her current position and her wet clothes. The nurse stands at the end of the bed and talks to the relative and explains that the woman's medical condition is under control and they are not concerned; otherwise she is there mainly for 'TLC' after her fall. The woman and her relative continue to say that she is uncomfortable in both her position and her wet nightie and sheets. The nurse says that other nurses will come along later and sort it out... more than an hour passes and nothing happens until the relative intervenes.

Meanwhile the patient opposite says she is extremely thirsty and asks for a drink. Care assistants leave a cup of tea but this is taken away by a nurse and replaced by a 'feeding' beaker of water with a straw. This is again left on a bed table at the side, out of reach of her arm which is entangled with intravenous lines and monitors. No assistance is given. She tries desperately to pick up the drinking beaker but can't. She cries about how thirsty she is. The visitor cannot look on without assisting and the woman expresses how grateful she is, evident in both her voice and her eyes.

The visitor is left shocked and bemused; how can what she is seeing be considered to be 'tender loving care'?

• Imagine yourself in the position of either (or both) of the patients described here. What aspects of care cause you concern?

What is apparent in the hypothetical case above is that care has both an instrumental component (the act of doing) and an affective component (the way in which the act is carried out; the attitudinal and emotional component of caring) (Watson, 2012, p.6).

You may have identified a number of aspects of therapeutic or clinical intervention. You might assume that various forms of clinical assessment took place in Accident and Emergency in order to diagnose heart failure and this continues to be assessed through observations and monitors; that medication has been prescribed and administered; that X-rays have been performed to rule out fractures; that the patient has been positioned on her side, perhaps as part of an assessment of risk of pressure sores.

The relative has no reason to doubt the technical, clinical and medical intervention. What seems to be absent is the affective and interpersonal dimension of care. There is an apparent lack of empathy and due regard for both women's distress and discomfort.

The nurse does not identify with their misplaced sense of self-blame and embarrassment for their mishaps and their feelings of inadequacy in the face of their sudden and unexpected admissions to hospital. Similarly there is little respect for the relative's well-founded concern and requests for assistance.

Good care is most often felt and experienced rather than understood intellectually; it is found in the positive emotional response to our interactions and gratitude for others' appreciation of our needs. Good care requires emotional intelligence and excellent communication and interpersonal skills in all their forms. As Tschudin (2003, p.7) points out, '... caring can only be experienced, and the quality of that experience is what matters'.

What is clearly evident here is the indifference and the lack of benevolence displayed and the total disregard for the women's comfort, their dignity and respect for their humanity. There is a disconnect between what is done (or not done), what is expressed and what might actually constitute good, 'loving' or kind care in this instance. It is insufficient to claim to be giving tender loving care if this is void of true meaning; an empty statement.

Tender 'loving' care is deeply rooted in relationship; the dynamic, interpersonal connection that exists between the carer and the 'cared for'. This comes from a real commitment to 'seek to sustain and elevate the welfare of another ... [for] ... to talk of loving in the absence of action is vacuous'. (Kendrick and Robinson, 2002, p.295). As Kendrick and Robinson (2002, p.292, 296) point out, 'loving' in this context is not simply sentimentalism. It involves commitment and affirms a sense of fidelity (faithfulness, trustworthiness) to the patient. It can include attentive listening to the patient's fears, gentle touch, conveying the sense that they matter to you and they are valued; interactions that are transformational, restorative and sustaining.

It is important to remember that although some of the incidents in the Francis Inquiry (Francis, 2010, 2013) and at Winterbourne View (DH, 2012b) were extreme acts of cruelty, many were not. Yet they were still very much felt by the patients, service users and relatives concerned. A practitioner does not have to be cruel to be without heart or compassion. Good care requires more than conscientiousness and working hard to fulfil our responsibilities or adhering to rules and principles; it is also about kindness. Kindness leads us to recognise the distress of another and to help them (Tong, 1998, pp.150–1).

Ballatt and Campling (2011, p.3) remind us that kinship and the way this is expressed through the compassionate relationship between a skilled carer and the person 'cared for', should be central to healthcare. To fail in this regard is to fail to address what makes people 'do well for others'. Having compassion may lead a person to show kindness towards others but it is possible to be kind without necessarily having or showing compassion. Thus, Ballatt and Campling (2011) view kindness in healthcare as requiring a particular intelligence for it to be both useful and wise. Again, this is not about sentimentality but about 'an intellectual and emotional understanding that self-interest and the interests of others are bound together...' (p.4). Intelligent kindness consists in acting on this understanding and promoting and protecting kindness and its attentiveness to others' needs, which in turn promotes wellbeing (Ballatt and Campling, 2011, pp.4–5).

This emotional appreciation and a notion of intelligent kindness are essential elements to an understanding of compassion in care.

COMPASSION IN CARE POLICY

We have already used the term 'compassion' several times as if there is some common shared understanding of compassion in care practice and that its moral value is taken for granted. Compassion has certainly been at the forefront of much debate in health and social care policy and practice in recent years, with the aim of putting compassion back into the heart of healthcare (DH, 2015a; DH 2012a, 2012b and 2012c; Dewar *et al.*, 2011; Firth-Cozens and Cornwell, 2009; Francis, 2010 and 2013; Parliamentary and Health Service Ombudsman, 2011; Youngson, 2008 and 2012).

Department of Health papers and reports claim to reinforce fundamental values of healthcare, including the expectation of compassionate care. For example, in *Front Line Care* (DH, 2010a, p.3), the Prime Minister's Commission recognised that true compassionate care '...is skilled, competent, value based care that respects individual dignity ... [and] ... requires the highest levels of skills and professionalism'. In response to failures in care identified through the Francis Inquiry (Francis, 2010 and 2013), the White Paper *Caring for our Future: reforming care and support* (DH, 2012a) and *Compassion in Practice for Nurses, Midwives and Care Staff* (DH and NHSCB, 2012c) emphasised the fundamental values of respect, dignity and compassion in care. This raised the expectation for all staff to deliver high quality, compassionate care and to treat people with care, dignity, respect and compassion.

The Royal College of Nursing (RCN, 2011a) identify eight principles of nursing practice, of which the first, 'Principle A – Dignity, humanity and equality' relates specifically to compassion. This forms an expectation for the starting point for care practice in all care settings as well as in all fields of nursing. It states:

> 'Nurses and nursing staff treat everyone in their care with dignity and humanity – they understand their individual needs, show compassion and sensitivity, and provide care in a way that respects all people equally.'
>
> (RCN, 2011a; Jackson and Irwin, 2011)

Similarly, the NHS Constitution (DH, 2015a) establishes the principles and values which should underpin the health service, including compassion as expressed by patients, public and staff. Thus patients should be able to expect this as an integral component of everyday care:

> 'We ensure that compassion is central to the care we provide and respond with humanity and kindness to each person's pain, distress, anxiety or need. We search for the things we can do, however small, to give comfort and relieve suffering. We find time for patients, their families and carers, as well as those we work alongside. We do not wait to be asked, because we care.'
>
> (DH, 2015a, p.5)

Yet, despite the undeniable focus on compassion, there are a number of challenges in the claims made for compassion in care. These include establishing a shared definition and understanding of the moral value of compassion, and then identifying what we mean by good compassionate care and how this can be promoted in care practice.

DEFINING COMPASSION

In defining compassion you may have used words like 'empathy', 'sympathy', 'pity', 'kindness', 'respect' and the need for appreciation of another's 'suffering'. Although pity, sympathy, empathy and compassion are similar emotions in that they are all 'other-regarding' and relate most often to the negative condition of another, they are also quite distinct in meaning.

Feeling pity involves feeling sorry for another but where we do not believe that we could or would have the same misfortune or have the negative experience in the same degrading or humiliating way. We can pity someone while maintaining an emotional distance from them. Thus, pity is sometimes seen as a negative emotion. In denying that we could experience the same misfortune, pity can involve some sense of superiority to the unfortunate and condescension, even that the person deserves the misfortune or has brought it on themselves (Blum, 1987, cited by Snow, 1991, p.196).

Sympathy differs from compassion in that it is an appropriate emotional response to a wide range of misfortunes but it does not demand a response. For example, we may feel sympathy for someone whose car has been scratched but, although we may believe this is unfortunate, we do not see it as a tragic event (Snow, 1991), neither does it entail any action on our part.

Empathy is a predominantly cognitive attribute that involves a deeper understanding of experiences, concerns and perspectives of another person, combined with a capacity to communicate this understanding (Hojat, 2009). For Crisp (2008, p.234), empathy consists in '…any kind of imaginative reconstruction of another's experience,

ACTIVITY 3.2

The meaning of compassion

1. What does compassion mean to you? Think about and write down your definition of 'compassion'.

2. If you find this difficult, create a concept map showing different words, phrases and ideas that come to mind when you think about 'compassion'.

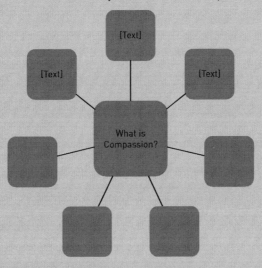

It might help to think about what a compassionate person might demonstrate in their relationship with others that the non-compassionate person might not.

Compassionate	Non-compassionate

3. Now talk to some relatives, friends and/or colleagues about their understanding of the term 'compassion'.

4. Try rewriting your definition now.

independently of any evaluation of it as good, bad, or indifferent'. Empathy implies a greater understanding of another person's reality but does not specifically require action. It is often viewed as the way into another person's emotions, with some other purpose or motive. The ability to '... perceive the meanings and feelings of another person and to communicate that understanding back to the person... can be a very influential mechanism for empowering that person.' (von Dietze and Orb, 2000, p.168).

Empathetic reconstruction can involve compassion but need not be a necessary condition for compassion. It is also possible, and often encouraged, to form empathetic yet professionally detached relationships with those in our care (von Dietze and Orb, 2000). This detachment is essentially incompatible with being compassionate which expects a deeper involvement in the suffering (or vulnerability) of another. Having empathy or sympathy need not imply good care or make claims on our motivations or behaviours. However, this is not to say that both are not desirable emotions for care practitioners; we should empathise with our patients or clients and this may elicit an appropriate response to a person's needs and lead to therapeutic intervention.

The word *compassion* is derived from the Latin words *com* (with) and *pati* (to suffer); thus literally compassion means 'to suffer with'. Compassion involves an intense emotional response of *'suffering with'* the other, analogous to the intensity of fear or anger (Crisp, 2008, p.235). Yet we tend to view compassion in a positive way; we like to think we are compassionate people and that this is a natural response to another's suffering. Compassion is also a morally significant emotion that includes an altruistic concern for another's good. Identifying with the other's plight through the belief that 'this could be me' enables you to put yourself in the place of the other and identify with their distress and suffering.

Compassion has a spiritual as well as philosophical origin. Karen Armstrong (2011), in her book *Twelve Steps to a Compassionate Life* and her work to develop a 'Charter for Compassion' (see the latest developments at charterforcompassion.org), aims to restore compassion as a fundamental virtue in religious and moral life. At the centre of the Charter, and beliefs about compassion, is the call to all humans to the imperative to apply the 'Golden Rule' (first identified by Confucius (551–479 BC)); *to ensure that all people are treated as we would wish to be treated ourselves.* Armstrong identifies that all the major religions place great importance on compassion, that compassion is inseparable from humanity and that '… instead of being motivated by self-interest, a truly humane person (is) consistently oriented to others'(Armstrong, 2011, p.7).

Compassion

> '…impels us to work tirelessly to alleviate the suffering of our fellow creatures, to dethrone ourselves from the centre of our world and put another there, and to honour the inviolable sanctity of every single human being, treating everybody, without exception, with absolute justice, equity and respect … Born out of deep interdependence, compassion is essential to human relationships and to a fulfilled humanity.'
> (extract from the Charter for Compassion 2009 in Armstrong, 2011, pp.4–5)

Thus, compassion is somewhat different from feeling pity, sympathy or empathy for another. It is not only about attending to suffering but recognising and responding to it (Snow, 1991). This last point is important in thinking about compassionate care, as not all acts need be in response to intense suffering to be distinguished as acts of compassion. 'Noticing potential vulnerability can be the precursor to compassionate behaviour…' (Dewar, 2013, p.3).

The combination of emotional response and deliberate action is evident in a number of definitions of compassion (see *Box 3.1*).

BOX — 3.1

Some definitions of compassion

The Oxford English Dictionary defines compassion as:

1. Suffering together with another, participation in suffering; fellow-feeling, empathy.

2. The feeling or emotion, when a person is moved by the suffering or distress of another, and by the desire to relieve it; pity that inclines one to spare or to succour.

3. Sorrowful emotion, sorrow, grief.' (OED, 1989, p.597)

'A deep awareness of the suffering of another coupled with a wish to relieve it.' (Chochinov, 2007, p.184)

'A relatively intense emotional response to the serious misfortune of another. The response is a "suffering with" the other and includes a concern for the other's good…' (Snow, 1991, p.197)

'Compassion is not a simple feeling state but a complex emotional attitude toward another, characteristically involving imaginative dwelling on the condition of the other person, an active regard for his good, a view of him as a fellow human being, and emotional responses of a certain degree of intensity.' Blum (1980, p.509)

'Compassion asks us to go where it hurts, to enter into places of pain, to share in brokenness, fear, confusion and anguish. Compassion challenges us to cry out with those in misery, to mourn with those who are lonely, to weep with those in tears. Compassion requires us to be weak with the weak, vulnerable with the vulnerable, and powerless with the powerless. Compassion means full immersion into the condition of being human.' (Nouwen *et al.*, 1982, p.4)

'A deep feeling of connectedness with the experience of human suffering that requires personal knowing of the suffering of others, evokes a moral response to the recognised suffering and that results in caring that brings comfort to the sufferer.' (Peters, 2006, p.39)

The philosopher Martha Nussbaum (2001, p.301) defines compassion as 'the painful emotion caused by the awareness of another person's undeserved misfortune…'. She identifies three moral emotional or cognitive requirements, based in the work of Aristotle, that are necessary for creation of compassion (Nussbaum, 2001, p.306):

- The 'seriousness requirement' – the harm suffered is significant rather than trivial.
- The 'desert requirement' – the misfortune is undeserved; it is not the person's fault.
- The 'similar possibilities requirement' – the suffering is something which could befall the person experiencing compassion (or someone close to her); it creates a painful emotion in us because we are also vulnerable to the misfortune.

We might question whether a person's misfortune has to be undeserved for you to feel compassion towards them. Certainly care needs to be taken in determining what may or may not be a person's 'own fault' and need not make them any less deserving of your respect. Nussbaum also amends the 'similar possibilities' requirement to acknowledge that we do not need to feel the same as the sufferer but should be able to understand their suffering from their perspective and recognise that this threatens their wellbeing and 'human flourishing'. We do not need a sense of fear but a sense of the other person's vulnerability in order to have compassion (Faust, 2009). Thus there is an emotional, cognitive and reflective element to compassion. Nussbaum goes on to acknowledge that sustained commitment to want to do something to relieve the suffering is what should motivate us to action (Nussbaum, 2001, p.399).

Martha Nussbaum (1996) also argues that compassion provides an important link between the interests of individuals and those of the community. Compassion is sometimes criticised as being an irrational force based in sentiment and emotion that may mislead or distract us when thinking about society and social policy. However, Nussbaum suggests that while compassion involves emotion, this should not be dismissed as it is also based in thought and evaluation about the wellbeing of others. If we want a compassionate community, we do not have to sacrifice reason and reflection because compassion involves another certain sort of deliberation and reasoning that leads to compassionate action.

THE VIRTUE OF COMPASSION

Although it is possible to see some valuable components in the definitions of compassion for understanding care practice, it is not the definition of compassion itself which has moral value. The moral value comes from the nature of compassion as a virtue; seeing compassion as part of our moral character, that is concerned with our and others' humanity and a number of human goods, including altruism. Aristotle, an ancient Greek philosopher, is viewed as one of the founding fathers of virtue ethics; where the key question is establishing what it means to 'live the good (or virtuous) life'. For Aristotle, being virtuous is a state involving rational choice and any virtue must concern action as well as feeling. So the compassionate person should not only feel compassion but also act compassionately (Crisp, 2008).

Drawing on Aristotle's approach to defining virtues, Crisp (2008) identifies the virtue of compassion consisting in having the disposition to feel compassion at the right time, about the right things, towards the right people, for the right end, and in the right way and without excess or deficiency. The excess is not about feeling too much compassion; it is not purely quantitative but about, for example, feeling compassion at the wrong time, for the wrong end. The deficiency of compassion (the vice of 'callousness') is often evident in reports of poor health and social care (Francis, 2013; PHSO, 2011).

Crisp (2008) goes on to give some examples of deficiency in compassion:

> 'Consider someone who fails to feel compassion when confronted by photographs of people suffering from some disaster. They are failing to feel as they should at the right time, at the right things, for the right people, and for the right end. And if perhaps they feel a slight twinge of compassion and nothing more, then they are failing to feel compassion in the right way ... Someone who shows condescending and inappropriate pity for the disabled feels compassion at the wrong time and towards the wrong people. In a case in which compassion for some disabled person is called for, but where the onlooker is feeling sorry for the person merely because of how they look (rather than because of the burdens imposed on them by how they look), then compassion is being felt for the wrong things and in the wrong way. Someone might feel compassion at the right time, for the right things, for the right people, and to the right degree, but do so because she enjoys the self-satisfaction she achieves through reflection on how kind she is being. So her compassion is felt for the wrong end or the wrong reason.'
>
> (Crisp, 2008, p.242)

Crisp's identification of the many reasons for potential deficiencies in being compassionate raises the need for caution in too easily claiming compassion as a value for healthcare or simply paying lip service to what this means and requires.

Beauchamp and Childress (2013, p.37) see compassion as one of five focal virtues for healthcare professionals that provide the practitioner's 'moral compass of character' (the others they identify are discernment, trustworthiness, integrity and conscientiousness). They define the virtue of compassion as combining:

'...an *attitude* of active regard for another's welfare with an *imaginative awareness and emotional response* of sympathy, tenderness, and discomfort at another's misfortune or suffering.' (Beauchamp and Childress, 2013, p.37, our emphasis).

Thus compassion has been viewed as the 'prelude to caring'; feeling compassion results in a caring response (Beauchamp and Childress, 2013, p.37). Being compassionate may be expressed in beneficent acts (acting kindly, to benefit) that aim to alleviate the misfortune or suffering of another. This will involve some degree of empathy for the person or persons concerned, which requires insights into their particular feelings and experiences of their illness, condition, disability, pain or suffering.

Being compassionate also requires the recognition of the uniqueness of another individual, the willingness to enter into a relationship with them and acting with a view to alleviating that person's suffering. This is clearly evident in Peters' (2006, p.39) definition of compassion, which identifies the centrality of emotions, the need to know the person, the moral dimension in the response to the person's suffering and incorporates the outcome of acting in a compassionate way, with reference to 'comforting'. Nouwen *et al.* (1982) view compassion as such an obvious reaction to human suffering that being accused of lacking compassion is almost synonymous with being accused of lacking humanity.

For von Dietze and Orb (2000, p.170) compassion as a virtue involves '…intentional, deliberate voluntary behaviour in support of another person that is not given with the expectation of any reward or punishment.'

Being compassionate requires shared experience and action as well as feelings. In a moment of crisis, a compassionate person will be physically present, will be there for the person and will offer consolation and support (Nouwen *et al.*, 1982). Thus, there is a tendency to think that feeling compassion is (nearly) always admirable (Crisp, 2008), although Beauchamp and Childress (2013, p.38) acknowledge that compassion may cloud clinical judgement and preclude rational and effective responses.

COMPASSIONATE CARE

Both compassion and caring are fundamental values that should be integral to the practice of health and social care. We have identified a number of the dimensions important to understanding compassionate care in the previous sections (these are summarised in *Box 3.2*). However, what compassionate care demands of the care practitioner and how this can be developed in practice need further exploration.

Although much is written about what it means to 'be compassionate', the practice of compassionate care is a more complex process. Compassion is found not only in the way actions are performed, the attitude and approach of the carer, but also in the level of consciousness and awareness of the others' suffering or pain. It starts from your ability to reflect on your 'self'; your thoughts, feelings and attitudes towards others and to consider the experience of care giving and care receiving. The emotional component of compassionate caring requires certain abilities to tolerate difficult feelings and situations as well as the more positive experiences. You will need to be emotionally attuned to yourself and others in your interactions and relationships (Dewar, 2013); try completing *Activity 3.3*.

BOX — **3.2**

Dimensions of compassionate care

- It is a subjective experience.
- It involves a caring moral attitude; knowing how to be, as much as how to act.
- It shows respect for the person and their humanity.
- It involves recognition of, and motivation to alleviate, suffering and vulnerability of others.
- It involves an affective response to the suffering and vulnerability of others, e.g. feelings of concern, sadness, kindness.
- It is person centred and relationship focused.
- It requires that practitioners acknowledge *the person* with the health need, illness or disability.
- It relates to the needs of others and demonstrates an active regard for the individual's good.
- It exists in the importance and quality of the relationships and interactions between individuals.
- It is about human experience and preserving the integrity of the individual.
- It requires emotional connection, real dialogue and excellent communication and interpersonal skills in all their forms.
- It requires action in response to the suffering or vulnerabilities of the other.

Adapted from Beauchamp and Childress, 2013; Blum, 1980; Dewar, 2013; von Dietze and Orb, 2000; Firth-Cozens and Cornwell, 2009; Schantz, 2007; Schulz, *et al.* 2007; Straughair, 2012b; Youngson, 2012.

Being compassionate has cognitive, emotional, and motivational components which are summarised by Schulz *et al.* (2007, p.6) in defining the compassionate individual, who:

> '... must be able to recognize and empathize with the person in distress, feel some connection toward the sufferer, experience both positive (e.g. love, concern) and negative (e.g. upset, distress about the suffering of another) affect, and be motivated to reduce or diminish that suffering.'

Compassionate care is not simply about alleviating a person's pain or suffering but about sharing the burden with them; compassion is not about '...what we choose to do *for* other people, but what we choose to do *together* with them' (von Dietze and Orb, 2000, p.169). Hence compassionate care should be both person centred and relationship focused (Dewar, 2011). Compassion involves both insight and thoughtfulness and emphasises emotional resonance; the active imagination of the sufferer's condition, concern for his or her good and a sense of sharing his or her distress (Blum, 1980).

ACTIVITY 3.3

Thinking compassionately

Identify three specific people that you know (friends, family, colleagues), to include:

- Someone for whom you have no particular strong feelings one way or another
- Someone you like, friend or family
- Someone you dislike.

For each, think about the following:

- Consider their good points, the contributions they make to your life
- Try to view each person as if you were 'in their shoes' or 'in their heart'. Can you identify any incidences of their pain or suffering? What could you do to alleviate or relieve this suffering? Think about this carefully; it may be particularly difficult for the person you do not like.
- What gets in the way of your compassion for the person you dislike?

Resolve to translate good thoughts about each of these individuals into small, concrete acts of friendship towards at least one of them.

Now repeat the activity but substitute the 'three people' for 'three patients', to include:

- A patient or client for whom you have no particular strong feelings one way or another
- A patient you like and enjoy caring for
- A patient you dislike or find difficult to care for.

Reflect on what gets in the way of your compassion for the patient you dislike or find difficult to care for.

What one small change could you make to your practice that would show positive compassionate regard for this patient?

Adapted from an approach to meditation in 'The Fourth Step – Empathy' of Armstrong's (2011) *Twelve Steps to a Compassionate Life.*

Gilbert (2009) identifies two different psychologies associated with being compassionate; one focuses on engagement and understanding, and the other on alleviation and relieving. The first approach, *'psychology of engagement and understanding'*, requires the ability and motivation to engage emotionally with the other's suffering and to attend to it. This entails toleration of the distress of both the other person and your own. It also requires empathy in understanding the source and nature of the suffering and then to be non-judgemental or uncondemning in your interactions. The second approach, the *'psychology of alleviation and relieving'*, focuses on how we seek to alleviate distress and suffering by being aware of and practising appropriate ways of thinking, feeling and behaving. These two approaches mutually influence each other. Gilbert refers to compassion as a '… social mentality because it integrates motivation, thinking, feeling, and behaviour in specific ways to achieve specific goals' (Gilbert, 2009, cited by Crawford et al., 2013, p.720).

Crawford et al. (2013) explored the language of 'compassionate mentality' as used by acute mental health practitioners, including psychiatrists, ward managers, nurses and healthcare assistants. The aim was to provide insights into practitioner perspectives of compassion in acute mental health and the ways in which threats ('threat stress') might influence their perspective on compassion. The practitioners interviewed did not describe compassion in their care and exhibited what was termed a 'production-line mentality' which appeared to pose a threat to their compassionate mentality. There was significantly heightened threat around managing and 'processing' patients to reach targets in the context of resources shortages, both of staffing and of time. In spite of their concern to deliver a quality service, the language used identified an institutional mentality and an emotional distancing between practitioners and patients. The researchers could not conclude that the practitioners were non-compassionate in their practice but they did demonstrate an obvious difficulty in articulating compassion. This was clearly linked to the 'threat stress' associated with the 'production-line' approach to care delivery. Thus there are wider organisational implications in creating a supportive culture of compassionate care (Francis, 2013; Youngson, 2008).

Being compassionate is not without difficulties for individual practitioners. The intense emotional implications and sequelae that can come from the close interpersonal relationships with patients and families in compassionate care has been described as 'compassion fatigue' (Austin et al., 2009; Aycock and Boyle, 2009; Walton and Alvarez, 2010). These sequelae can include burnout, traumatic stress disorder, indirect traumatisation, victimisation, compassion stress and emotional contagion (feeling and expressing emotions similar to and influenced by those of others, including their negative thoughts and anxieties) (Austin et al., 2009).

Although these psychological and emotional implications of compassion have been identified in research related to health and care practitioners, they need not be unique to formal caring roles and may be experienced by lay carers, family and friends; anyone who is in an intense, sustained care relationship. Figley (1995, p.1) described the 'cost of caring' (or compassion fatigue) as a form of secondary traumatic stress disorder where empathetic caregivers indirectly experience the fear, pain and suffering of their patients (or relatives) and some loss of their own sense of self. Thus, it is important to be conscious of the ways in which you might internalise other people's suffering. However, this in itself is not a reason to avoid compassionate care and as Dewar (2013) reminds us, compassionate caring need not be an emotional burden but a privilege that brings positive reward and job satisfaction in the delivery of good care.

THE EXPERIENCE OF COMPASSIONATE CARE

Local research with a group of service users and 'lay' carers identified what they saw as essential features of good care (Quallington, 2011). These are summarised as:
- Kind, caring and compassionate
- Competent
- Emotionally intelligent, able to communicate and respond effectively
- Loyal and dependable
- Responsible
- Self-motivating and having initiative
- Puts patient/individual first
- Positive attitude and willingness to help.

The most notable thing about this list is that the most important features of care for recipients are those that relate to good human interaction which are key to compassionate care and not the technical, clinical skills. Although competent and skilled practice is both expected and necessary, these features do not take precedence in defining good care. What is clear from both this small-scale research and the wider evidence is that kindness and compassion are viewed as fundamental for the experience of good care.

Drawing on her doctoral work, Dewar (2013, p.50) provides a useful summary of the key elements of care that are valued by patients and contribute to their experience of good compassionate care. These include patients or service users:
- Being able to freely express emotions such as suffering and vulnerability
- Being valued and having individual needs recognised
- Being given choice and opportunities to be involved in care and decision-making
- Being respected
- Being cared for by kind, warm and genuine staff
- Being given time by healthcare professionals
- Being given information by staff.

Similarly, the Association for Improvements in the Maternity Services (AIMS, 2012) identified what women want from their midwife in the woman-centred care relationship which reflects a number of dimensions of compassionate care; see *Box 3.3*.

There is much to be learned for compassionate care from the philosophy of woman-centred care in midwifery (and from feminist relational approaches to understanding

> **BOX 3.3**
>
> **Top ten tips – what women want from their midwife**
> - Listen to women
> - Be an advocate for women
> - Understand informed decision-making
> - Respect women
> - Value your skills in normal birth
> - Be a courageous professional
> - Work collaboratively
> - Use positive body language
> - Know when to be silent
> - Be engaged and humane.
>
> (excerpt from AIMS, 2012)

autonomy; see *Chapter 6*). The fundamental role of the midwife in her relationship with the woman is:

> '... to watch, to listen and to respond to any given situation with all [their] senses... the conscious and subconscious knowing ... knowing when to inform, suggest, act, seek help and, most importantly, be still or withdraw.'
>
> (Leap, 2000, p.5).

Siddiqui (1999, pp.111–13) identifies key components essential to this therapeutic relationship of midwifery that are based in deep, meaningful and highly developed communication and interpersonal skills and in a virtue-based ethics of care. There is the need for a caring moral conscience, commitment, compassion and empathy coupled with insight into their own being and providing a *'presence'*. A sense of being in contact with the thoughts and spirit of the woman at the heart of the relationship is required, rather than being present but emotionally and spiritually detached, as is a demonstrating of the value of respect for persons through an empowering relationship of '...mutual understanding, awareness of each other and a recognition of the full potential of the woman'. (Siddiqui, 1999, p.113). Thus, the relationship between the midwife and woman is seen as crucial (Guilliland and Pairman, 1995; Leap, 2000; Kennedy *et al.*, 2004), as is developing self-trust and mutual trust between the woman and the midwife in a caring relationship (McLeod and Sherwin, 2000; McLeod 2002). Page (2003, p.119) declares the midwife–woman relationship to be 'the crux of effective, sensitive, and autonomous care'. This philosophy of care would sit well with a more universal vision of compassionate care.

Van der Cingel's research (see van der Cingel 2009; 2011; 2014) into the experiences and views of compassion of nurses and older people with chronic disease identified seven dimensions of compassion that inform the qualities and skills needed in compassionate caring (see *Box 3.4*).

BOX — 3.4

Qualities and skills for compassionate care

Attentiveness: consciously showing interest in whatever issue is important to the other person in the person-to-person encounter; approaching them as a fellow human being.

Active listening: inviting and stimulating the patient to 'tell their story'; using silences and questioning to encourage sharing of emotions.

Naming of suffering: identifying the emotional significance of the patient's suffering and confronting them with this; acknowledging the person's suffering as a visible aspect of life rather than something to be concealed; reassuring the patient that these feelings and emotions are rightly felt. Use paraphrasing of what you hear and value the patient's situation as feeling unpleasant, difficult, tedious or bad *for them*.

Involvement: mutuality that comes from showing that the patient's predicament touches and resonates with you; trusting that the emotion shared with you will be safe.

Helping: practical component of compassion; anticipating needs and helping in a variety of ways.

Being present: a physical as well as emotional presence; to notice what is most important for the patient and to be there when needed; a conscious choice and alertness to notice what is necessary.

Understanding: the suffering and emotions that go with the person's suffering and associated loss; checking whether your interpretation is correct; the human thing to do; professional behaviour using an inquiring attitude leads to personal knowledge about the patient that establishes the right goals and outcomes of care for that patient.

Adapted from van der Cingel's (2014, p.1255) seven dimensions of compassion.

Well-developed communication and interpersonal skills as well as real insight into the person are therefore key to practising compassionate care. Firth-Cozens and Cornwell (2009, p.3) see this as more than 'good' communication and requiring 'real dialogue' which sees the whole person in the patient. Real dialogue '… is spoken human to human rather than clinician to patient; it shows interest; never stereotypes but recognises and enjoys difference while also appreciating the common core of humanity; it includes honesty where necessary, and may need courage at times.'

Morse *et al.* (1992, 2006) reviewed therapeutic communication strategies and proposed an alternative communication model based in an understanding of empathy. Therapeutic communication strategies used in clinical practice with patients who are suffering are identified, and the communication process of emotive engagement or embodiment as reflected in the interactions that occur between caregivers and patients is illustrated. This model is based on two broad characteristics:

1. whether the nurse is focused on the patient's response (i.e. engaged and, therefore, embodying the sufferer's experience) or focused on the self, protecting him-/herself from experiencing the patient's suffering, and

2. whether the response is reflexive and spontaneous (first-level) or learned (second-level) and, therefore, controlled.

The relationship between the four categories of responses identified by Morse *et al.* (2006, p.77, Figure 4) are shown in *Figure 3.2.* The proposed model extends previously limited models of empathy and provides insight into non-therapeutic as well as therapeutic responses.

		FOCUS		
	Sufferer-focused (patient)		Self-focused (professional)	
	CHARACTERISTIC	RESPONSE	RESPONSE	CHARACTERISTIC
First-level	Engaged (with sufferer's emotion) Genuine Reflexive	Pity Sympathy Consolation Commiseration Compassion Reflexive reassurance	Guarding Shielding/steeling/ bracing Dehumanising Withdrawing Distancing Labelling Denying	Anti-engaged (against embodiment; protective)

Second-level	Pseudo-engaged
	
	Learned
	Professional
		Sharing self
		Humour
		Reassurance
		  (informing)
		Therapeutic empathy
		Confronting
		Comforting
		  (learned)
			Rote behaviours
			  'professional style'
			Legitimising/justifying
			Pity
			  (false/professional)
			Stranger
			Reassurance (false)
				A-engaged
				
				(embodiment absent
				or removed)

Figure 3.2 *Types of responses by focus and experience of caregiver. Reproduced from Morse* et al. *(2006, p.77, Fig. 4) with permission from John Wiley & Sons. "A-engaged" – a form of disengagement.*

From this typology, good compassionate care would require moving between the 'Second-level and First-level, Sufferer-focused' orientation in care. Thus the practitioner would be reflexive and demonstrate characteristics of genuineness and true engagement with the patient's emotional response to their own suffering rather than exhibiting learned, rote behaviours. It is perhaps easier to imagine providing this kind of care in a more sustained, one-to-one care relationship such as those previously described in midwifery or in palliative care, where there are excellent examples of compassion in care.

Part of the challenge for this approach in modern healthcare is the often transitory and fragmented nature of the patient or service user experience, particularly in the acute setting. However, Youngson (2008, 2012) claims that we should not use time as an excuse for not aiming to provide compassionate care and that this can be achieved through the simplest of interactions. He gives the example of a nurse 'minding the bumps' in a corridor by gently manoeuvring the trolley when transferring his daughter (who had a spinal injury) between departments. To Youngson, this simple action demonstrated real kindness, concern and understanding for his daughter's suffering and needs; a compassionate response. In particular, he identifies the need to hone healthcare practitioners' communication and relationship skills:

> 'In today's pressured healthcare environment, we cannot afford to wait days to learn what our patients really need… it is possible to build trust in minutes and to get to the heart of concerns in the course of one visit… Empathy is as much a skill as an inborn character trait.'
>
> (Youngson, 2008, p.4).

Recent doctoral work by Belinda Dewar (2011) captures the notion of the importance of relationships and relational knowledge in compassionate care and identifies ways in which compassionate, relationship-centred care can be implemented in practice. Dewar and Nolan's (2013) study in an older people care setting demonstrates that even the most transient of contacts can reflect supportive connection between those involved through engaging in 'appreciative caring conversations' (Dewar and Nolan, 2013).

ACTIVITY 3.4

'Appreciative Caring Conversations' for compassionate care

Locate a copy of the following article by Belinda Dewar and Mike Nolan:

Dewar, B. and Nolan, M. (2013) Caring about caring: developing a model to implement compassionate relationship centred care in an older people care setting. *International Journal of Nursing Studies*, 50(9): 1247–58.

Read the article with the following questions in mind and make key notes (it helps to read with a purpose)

1. What are the key attributes of a definition of compassion?
2. What types of relational knowledge underpin the notion of compassion and how is such knowledge established?
3. What are the 7 Cs of 'appreciative caring conversations'?
4. What are the benefits of this approach in caring for older people and how can care practitioners encourage such conversations?

BOX — 3.5

Questions to use in caring conversations with patients to engage them in compassionate, therapeutic relationships

Ask patients:

- What is important to you?
- Can you help me to understand what would help comfort you now?
- What else could we do to improve your experience?

Adapted from Dewar *et al.*, 2014.

A CULTURE OF COMPASSIONATE CARE

Robert Francis QC, in his report of the Mid Staffordshire NHS Foundation Trust Public Inquiry (Francis, 2013), concluded that in addition to safety, healthcare needs to have a culture of caring, commitment and compassion. On his account, this 'caring culture' is concerned with:

- Acceptance that patients' needs come before one's own
- Recognition of the need to empathise with patients and other service users
- A willingness to provide patients and other service users with the assistance that one would want for oneself, or to refer them to a person with the ability to provide that help
- A willingness to listen to patients and service users to discover what they want for themselves
- A willingness to work together with others for the benefit of patients and other service users
- A commitment to draw concerns about patient safety and welfare to the attention of those who can address those concerns.

(Francis, 2013, p.1360, para. 20.12)

The appalling nature of some of the failings in care described in this inquiry cannot be denied. However, Youngson (2014) questions whether policy and regulation are the best approach to ensuring and implementing compassionate care. We also need to be careful not to rush to respond to crises in care and any associated government targets without first reflecting on the whole experience. As Gallagher reminds us,

> '... a kind of monomania results when individual concepts such as "dignity" and "compassion" are unreflectively embraced and inadequately applied. Individual practitioners may be blamed for care deficits rather than a nurse manager taking time to understand the complex mix of individual, organisational and political and social factors.'

Gallagher (2012, p.712).

Francis clearly identified failings and need for action at all levels of the organisation from individual care through to management, leadership and Government, as indicated by the 192 recommendations for change and service improvement. However, the question remains, how can we create and deliver a culture of compassionate care?

Youngson (2008 and 2012) views the alignment of policy, leadership and practice as being critical to putting compassion and care back into healthcare and in making a real difference to the patient's experience of 'being cared for'. However, this requires action at a variety of levels; in healthcare systems, by organisational leaders and by individuals. Youngson proposes an action plan for compassion in healthcare (Youngson, 2008, p.3) which includes:

- The declaration of 'compassion' as a core value for healthcare
- To seek to reward rather than punish those who practise compassionate caring and to allow time to care
- To improve communication and interpersonal skills, to take time to listen, develop trusting relationships and learn what patients really need
- To provide safe space for staff to have deep, meaningful, open conversations and discuss difficult issues, including personal vulnerability and fears
- To challenge models of professionalism that require rational detachment from those in our care and adopt humanistic approaches that strengthen empathy and capacity for compassionate caring
- To 'hard wire' compassionate behaviour into everyday practice, e.g. practise empathetic communication
- To declare compassion as a management and leadership competence; how patients experience care is a reflection of how the organisation treats its staff. Leaders should model compassionate behaviours found in person-centred care, be deeply respectful, humane and compassionate, celebrate diversity, listen deeply, be open, have integrity and not be afraid to say sorry
- Engage health consumers in the change – using the power of patient and service user experiences and narratives to open the hearts of practitioners and recognise the (negative) impact of cold detachment and the gratitude for compassionate caring.

Dewar *et al.* (2014) draw on their action research project 'Leadership in Compassionate Care Programme' in establishing key implications for the practice and education of compassionate care. They identify the need to review perceptions, practice and organisational infrastructures that support compassionate care and support development of the following in respect to individual practitioners, teams and organisations (Dewar *et al.*, 2014, pp.7–8):

- Identifying and articulating compassionate care practice in healthcare settings, including 'the small acts that matter'
- Celebrating and valuing compassionate care practices
- Creating working environments where relational approaches to care are encouraged

- Working with patients to check out what matters to them as individuals and using this information to influence care giving
- Incorporating caring conversations into daily work
- Organisational support enabling staff to experience fulfilment in giving compassionate care
- Supporting staff to engage in the practice of self-compassion
- Organisations supporting staff to maintain a focus on the development of compassionate care.

ACTIVITY 3.5

Access and read the article by Dewar, B. *et al.* (2014) Clarifying misconceptions about compassionate care. *Journal of Advanced Nursing*, 70(8): 1738–47.

- Establish why each of these dimensions of practice has been identified as important for delivering compassionate care.
- Think about what each element means in relation to your practice and care environment.
- Talk to your line manager and other members of your care team. What one small change could you make that would maximise impact for establishing, maintaining and enhancing compassionate care in your practice?

You may find it helpful to access some of Robin Youngson's work. For example, read *Time to Care* (Youngson, 2012) or his short paper, 'Compassion in Healthcare: the missing dimension of healthcare reform?' (Youngson, 2008). For a practical approach to identifying ways to strengthen compassion in healthcare, see Youngson (2014) where he outlines a workshop approach utilising appreciative inquiry. You could also look at the website 'Hearts in Healthcare' (heartsinhealthcare.com) created by Youngson as part of his work in 'rehumanising healthcare' and emphasising the power of healing relationships.

CONCLUSION

The value of compassion in care comes from the ways in which being compassionate emphasises the humane nature of caring in response to a person's vulnerabilities and suffering, the affective and emotional aspects of care and the importance of intelligent kindness. Being compassionate may be an inbuilt virtue, but understanding what it means to be compassionate, practising related skills and reflecting critically on our own and others' practice can lead to compassionate behaviour and action in care. This requires excellent communication and interpersonal skills, emotional intelligence, willingness to engage in appreciative, empathetic caring conversations and the need to build trusting, person-centred care relationships. What is clear is that compassion is insufficient as the only value for good care, which also requires, amongst others, due respect for humanity, for the individual person and their dignity.

CHAPTER SUMMARY

Eight key points to take away from Chapter 3:

- 'Good' care requires not only 'knowing-that' and 'knowing-how' but also demands a commitment to the caring process and a caring attitude.

- Caring behaviour fundamental to good care is found in the integration of competence, reasoning and judgement, a 'virtuous attitude' of caring and good moral character.

- Good care is most often felt and experienced rather than understood intellectually. It requires certain dispositions, such as patience, honesty, sensitivity, kindness and compassion, as well as practising according to a set of values, including respect, autonomy, honesty, trustworthiness and fairness.

- Caring attitudes and behaviours can alleviate human suffering and make a positive difference to a person's sense of wellbeing.

- Compassion is a morally significant emotion that includes an altruistic concern for another's good, putting yourself in the place of others and identifying with their distress and suffering (other-regarding).

- Being compassionate requires a combination of the emotional response and a virtuous attitude with deliberate action through recognising, responding and attending to the suffering of others.

- Compassionate care should respect the person and their humanity and be both person centred and relationship focused; it requires attentiveness, active listening and excellent communication and interpersonal skills, being present and understanding the person's suffering, anticipating needs and helping in a variety of ways.

- Both compassion and caring are fundamental values that should be integral to the practice of health and social care and realised through a culture of compassionate care.

FURTHER READING

Dewar, B. (2013) Cultivating compassionate care. *Nursing Standard*, **27(34):** 48–55.

Sellman, D. (2011) *What Makes a Good Nurse? Why the virtues are important for nurses.* London: Jessica Kingsley.

Straughair, C. (2012b) Exploring compassion: implications for contemporary nursing. Part 2, *British Journal of Nursing*, **21(4):** 239–244.

Youngson, R. (2012) *Time to Care. How to love your patients and your job.* New Zealand: Rebelheart Publishers.

04

RIGHTS, EQUALITY AND ANTI-DISCRIMINATORY PRACTICE

LEARNING OUTCOMES:

In this chapter you will:

- be introduced to the notion of rights and obligations

- focus on rights relevant to care practice

- examine the concepts of equality and anti-discriminatory practice

- reflect on strategies that can be employed to support and uphold rights in care practice.

INTRODUCTION

Beliefs about individual value and respect for others are central considerations in modern, western, democratic societies. The principle of respect for others is a consequence of the belief that individuals, just because they are individuals, are of value. The value of individuals is not attributed to them because of their role or position in society, or because of their achievements; rather it is because they are a person (this will be explored further in *Chapter 5*). The valuing of personhood in western societies affords us certain rights or entitlements that are not afforded to other species. However, accepting that individuals have rights also requires us to accept a concept of obligation, i.e. obligations that are owed in order to ensure that conditions exist in which rights can be upheld. This chapter will examine rights in the context of care services and will discuss how practitioners can help to support and promote others' rights. A section on rights has been included in this text because the values that are articulated and promised by practitioners, and expected by clients, are often claimed as rights. Rights claims are often evident in situations when individuals feel that they are not receiving the care to which they believe they are entitled. Rights values such as fairness, respect, dignity, equality and autonomy underpin the public service ethos, the NHS Constitution 2010 and many professional codes. However, things can sometimes go wrong and rights values can be infringed. For example, the European Nutrition for Health Alliance (2012) (european-nutrition.org/index.php/homestatistics) gained statistics from the Office of National Statistics to show that over 1300 people died of malnutrition or dehydration whilst in care in NHS or private hospitals in the preceding year, even though food and hydration are essential to sustain life. Failing to provide these basics to someone in your care, it could be argued, is a breach of their right to life.

Rights and values are thus intrinsically connected.

We live in a society in which we enjoy a multitude of rights, many of which are protected in law. In our day-to-day lives we are normally able to ensure that our rights are respected; and when we feel that our rights have been infringed we have the opportunity to raise a challenge. However, when individuals come into contact with care services it is easy for rights to be unwittingly infringed. Individuals may lack confidence in asserting their rights. When experiencing care, individuals may find themselves in environments outside of their normal experience, which impacts on their sense of personal control. Due to illness they may be feeling vulnerable, frail, in pain, frightened, bewildered, confused, out of their depth or simply lacking knowledge about their situation. In such situations a key responsibility of care practitioners is to recognise this, to understand what rights individuals are entitled to, to uphold these, to challenge any infringement and to support individuals to gain and maintain appropriate personal control and independence. Seedhouse (1998) asserts that the way that we treat those who are most vulnerable in our society is a reflection of the moral state of that society. We should be concerned about others' rights, particularly those who are most vulnerable, because it affirms their value.

ACTIVITY 4.1

- Can you think of a situation in which you felt that your rights were not respected?
- How did this make you feel?
- How did that impact on your behaviour?
- On reflection was the challenge to your rights justified or unjustified?

WHAT ARE RIGHTS?

Rights and the importance of their protection became firmly embedded in western society following the revelations of the mass violation of human rights that occurred during the Second World War; it generated a determination that this should never happen again. The notion of rights builds on the strongly-held belief that individuals are unique and intrinsically valuable; as a consequence they should be accorded respect and the entitlements that arise from that value. Focusing on rights enables us to explore issues from the point of view of the vulnerable rather than from the perspective of those in power who traditionally make the rules (Almond, 1993). That is to say, it allows us to examine the impact on, and implications for the recipient.

Rights are entitlements; something to which you are entitled without qualification.

Rights are not the same as privileges. Privileges are benefits that are offered but which can be withdrawn, because they are not recognised as entitlements. For example, in an overcrowded train you may be offered the privilege of sitting in the first class compartment of the train if there are spare seats, even if you only have a second class ticket. However, this is not a right and you could legitimately be asked to move.

- Unlike a privilege, an entitlement is something that it is generally agreed that an individual can reasonably expect to access. The right or entitlement may be as a 'valid claim'. It is helpful to see rights in terms of valid claims because it reminds us that in exercising our rights we are often claiming something from someone else. This chapter will focus mainly on the idea of rights as claims, but there are other definitions of rights.
- Rights are sometimes expressed as 'powers', for example, the legal power to determine what happens to your property after your death.
- Rights may also be expressed as immunities. Immunities are protections from the actions of another. For example, sex discrimination legislation protects women from an exploitative employer, who may wish to pay women less than men (Almond, 1993).

As a citizen, society affords us a number of rights or entitlements that support a valid claim from the State. For example: I have the right to access free education up to the age of 18; I have the right to vote, once I reach the age of majority; and I have the right to receive free healthcare. While I have the rights to make these claims, the right to these things is not without boundaries. Access to free healthcare is a reasonable, or valid, claim, given that Britain has a National Health Service (NHS), paid for by direct taxation. However, because the NHS is subject to limited resources, my right to receive healthcare is not unlimited. My right to receive healthcare must be balanced against the rights of others to receive healthcare. The conditions of 'valid' and 'reasonable' claims are important in the context of rights. It would not be reasonable for me to claim numerous, unnecessary, plastic surgery operations in an effort to make myself look better, if this was at the expense of someone else's right to claim life-saving treatment. It is, therefore, a valid claim to seek necessary treatment but not to seek unnecessary treatment.

DIFFERENT KINDS OF RIGHTS

Claim rights or entitlements are sometimes termed 'positive rights'. These rights require society, or another individual, to do something positive in order to fulfil or uphold the rights. For example, my claim for healthcare can only be realised if society ensures that healthcare systems exist for me to access healthcare, and if individuals in those systems fulfil their duty to provide me with the necessary care.

Human rights

These rights have been agreed by an international community as being the rights that any human is entitled to by virtue of them being human. Many societies protect these through the legal system but, when they are challenged, they may also be protected through the international community. For example, the international community may intervene by diplomacy or by force when human rights are being contravened. The Universal Declaration of Human Rights (1948) and the European Convention on Human Rights (1953) set out the rights that should be afforded to any individual by virtue of being human. These rights are protected in law and articulated in Britain through the Human Rights Act (1998) (see *Box 4.1*). When these rights are violated a citizen has the right to challenge this violation and, where relevant, seek appropriate action or compensation.

BOX 4.1

The Human Rights Act (1998)

The Human Rights Act (1998) sets out 16 basic rights that all people in Britain should enjoy:

1. The right to life (Article 2)
2. Prohibition of torture (Article 3)
3. Prohibition of slavery and forced labour (Article 4)
4. Right to liberty and security (Article 5)
5. Right to a fair trial (Article 6)
6. No punishment without law (Article 7)
7. Right to respect for private and family life (Article 8)
8. Freedom of thought, conscience and religion (Article 9)
9. Freedom of expression (Article 10)
10. Right to freedom of assembly and association (Article 11)
11. The right to marry (Article 12)
12. Prohibition of discrimination (Article 14)
13. Protection of property (Article 1 of Protocol 1)
14. Right to education (Article 2 of Protocol 1)
15. Right to free elections (Article 3 of Protocol 1)
16. Abolition of the death penalty (Article 1 of Protocol 6).

A number of these rights are more relevant to the health and care context than others. Since the Human Rights Act (1998) became operational in 2001 a number of cases have been brought to court. For example, the prohibition of torture has been used to bring cases against local authorities who failed to protect children from abuse. The right to liberty is relevant to the detention of individuals under the Mental Health Act (2007). Freedom from discrimination for those with a disability is also protected by the Equality Act 2010 (HMSO, 2010).

Legal rights

Legal rights are those rights that are enshrined in law and that society seeks to uphold by promise and through the justice system when these rights are challenged. For example, there is a legal right to equal pay for the same job.

Moral rights

Moral rights are rights that are associated with the manner in which people are treated. These rights may be identified through explicit public declarations of values and behaviours such as in professional codes, or they may be culturally assumed through the adoption of belief and value systems, such as the adoption of particular religious doctrines. These rights are much harder to protect as they are not clearly defined and are not always shared by everyone.

Negative rights or liberty rights

Negative or liberty rights do not require an individual to make a claim, nor to require another to provide something or do something. A negative right relates to the freedom to do something without interference. For example, the freedom of speech, the right to practise one's preferred religion (or the right not to practise a religion).

LIMITATIONS ON RIGHTS

It is important to recognise that, although rights are an important consideration in our culture, rights are rarely absolute and rights can be curtailed. If, in exercising my right to freedom of speech, I override others' rights by making sexist or racist remarks, I can have my right to freedom of speech legally curtailed. The curtailment only applies to those remarks that are in breach of anti-discriminatory laws and does not apply to my freedom of speech generally. This is a justified infringement of my rights. If, however, my rights are 'violated', this is an 'unjustified' infringement of my rights. For example, if I decide that I do not want to take part in a research project, but contrary to my wishes I am given the trial treatment without me realising, my right to refuse treatment and my right of informed consent will have been violated. The important point to note here is that at times, usually in extreme circumstances, rights can be infringed. However, when rights are infringed, it is important that that infringement can be justified robustly.

ACTIVITY 4.2

Can you think of any examples of justified infringements of rights in your care context?

You may have considered treatment without consent in an emergency situation, or treatment under the Mental Health Act for those displaying psychotic symptoms.

Can you justify these infringements?

RIGHTS IN CARE

Patient and service user rights in the care context are afforded to citizens by the State. They are clearly articulated in general patients' charters, in documents outlining rights for specific groups, for example, *NHS Treatment – Your Rights* (Rethink Mental Illness, 2017), or are articulated through the duties and responsibilities of care practitioners in their codes of practice (see HCPC Standards of Conduct, Performance and Ethics (HCPC, 2016) and *The Code* for nurses and midwives (NMC, 2015)). Rights are also articulated in legislation (e.g. Health and Social Care Act (2012); NHS Constitution (DH, 2015a)) and in the publication of national standards of service.

Rights, needs and wants

It is important to distinguish between 'rights', 'needs' and 'wants'. Public expectations are often confused between what the public would like, and believe they need, and what they are entitled to. Wants are often expressed in terms of rights as it is believed that, articulated in this way, they will have more legitimacy. It is important for the care practitioner to be able to differentiate between reasonable and justified needs and entitlements, and unjustified wants.

A need is a requirement. It is something where it can be demonstrated that the individual will suffer a significant harm if they are denied it (Doyal and Gough, 1991). A want is something that an individual would like, and which might even be desirable to provide, if the resources are available. However, a want is neither an entitlement nor a requirement; therefore, it should not be provided over the entitlements or needs of others.

As discussed earlier in the chapter, a right is something to which one is entitled. This may apply universally or be restricted to a specific group. In care provision entitlements to care may be justified in respect of level of need; the greater the need, the greater the entitlement to the provision. This enables those with more severe needs to make a stronger claim to have their needs met. Consequently, in an accident and emergency department the individual who has suffered a major trauma should take precedence over the minor sports injury. However, it is important to recognise that in a universal healthcare system, even minor injuries need treatment – the severity merely acts as a method for prioritising.

ACTIVITY 4.3

Make a list of the rights that you think people in your care should be entitled to and identify why you think these rights should be upheld.

Your list might include some of those identified in the rest of this chapter.

The right to be treated with respect and dignity

This principle was articulated in the 1994 Declaration on the Promotion of Patient Rights in Europe and is the basis for national laws and charters on service user and patient rights. Dignity and respect are key concepts in care. It is based on the belief that illness and vulnerability are not reasons to be treated less well than other people.

ACTIVITY 4.4

Think about how a person's respect and dignity can be eroded in a care environment.

- A person may have surrendered their clothes and been dressed in a thin gown that gapes at the back.
- The staff may have decided to try to be friendly by addressing someone by their first name, without checking how someone would prefer to be addressed.
- Whilst being assisted to wash, several people come behind the curtains to ask the carer questions.
- A healthcare professional assisting someone with their meal while holding a conversation with other staff or while looking at their phone.

While these are seemingly small transgressions they are quite significant in impacting on one's dignity. Think of ten examples of your own of how a person's dignity can be eroded.

Definitions of respect and dignity

Even though an individual may find themselves in a vulnerable or dependent situation they are entitled to the same level of dignity, respect and protection that can be expected by anyone in that society. This right is justified on grounds of our shared humanity.

The fact that we are all human means that no one is entitled to more, or less, dignity and respect than others.

Dignity and respect, like many commonly used terms in care, do not have a simple definition, but they can be broadly defined as being 'worthy of self-esteem' and having the 'esteem of others'. Seedhouse and Gallagher (2002) link dignity and respect to our capabilities and the opportunity to exercise those capabilities effectively. This definition helps us understand the concepts – think about how you feel when your dignity is infringed, or when your capabilities are compromised or thwarted by another. Lack of respect and dignity may leave us feeling devalued, worthless, frustrated and angry because it is a fundamental assault on the individual as a human. Care practitioners, through their work, are invited to be involved in intimate aspects of others' lives. They may be engaged in physically caring or be privy to personal affairs, such as financial information, family relationships, knowledge of personal needs and so on. People in receipt of care, by necessity, have less opportunity to maintain their privacy than others. This detailed knowledge of others could be a reason why dignity, privacy and respect are infringed. Over-familiarity, thinking that you know better than the person themselves about what is good for them, and the uninvited sharing of information with others are all examples of how care practitioners can infringe the rights and dignity of those in their care, even though this may be done with the best intentions. Care that respects dignity must be sensitive to the feelings and needs and rights of others in order that they can enjoy, as near as possible, the same level of respect and privacy as those not in receipt of care. Care workers must therefore develop sensitivity and good communication skills so that they can detect and interpret others' feelings, listen attentively to their needs and to communicate necessary information effectively in a manner that does not patronise or dictate.

We will discuss respect and dignity in more detail in *Chapter 5*.

ACTIVITY 4.5

Reflect on your own approach to the care of others. Tick as many of the words in the lists below that best reflect your beliefs and approach to care and discuss this with a colleague.

Support	Protect
Listen	Help
Consult	Risk
Partnership	Compliance
Educate	Inform
Independence	Responsibility
Equality	Persuade

A paternalistic approach to care

All of the words in the two lists above reflect appropriate attitudes to care. However, different approaches to care need to be used selectively and sensitively. If you ticked more words in the second column you may have a more protective or 'paternalistic' approach to care. When people feel particularly vulnerable a paternalistic approach to care can be the most appropriate because it relieves the stress and responsibility of decision-making. However, it is not normally desirable to sustain this approach to care, except when someone is progressively debilitated. In a 'paternalistic' relationship power resides with the caregiver. This creates a dependent relationship in which the recipient relies heavily on the care practitioner and which compromises the ability to assert rights and wishes that differ from the care practitioner's own perspective. The danger of this approach to care is that it does not create an environment in which the recipient can develop, take risks or become independent. If the carer persuades the recipient into a unwanted course of action they have not respected the individual's right to dignity. A paternalistic approach might be appropriate at times when an individual requires more than average support, due to their being 'more than ordinarily vulnerable' (Sellman, 2011 p.49). However, such an approach should be administered with caution to ensure that the support and protection offered by this approach to care do not inadvertently become unnecessarily controlling.

A care facilitator

If your approach reflected words mainly in the first column, you may be primarily someone who facilitates care and works collaboratively with the recipient, rather than controls care, i.e. someone who supports others to lead their own lives in their own way. You are adopting an approach that recognises the dignity, individuality and autonomy of the recipient. While this approach to care encourages independence and personal development, there is a danger that this may fail to protect the vulnerable person adequately. It can also bring the carer and patient into conflict as care recipients are at times reluctant to take responsibility and make choices. Sometimes those being cared for make what can be perceived as poor choices, which could leave the care worker feeling frustrated or angry. As long as the patient has received relevant information on which to make their choice, even poor choices should be accepted. Evidence tells us that smoking is a poor health choice but it is still a legal right to make that choice. It is only restricted when it impinges on others' right to have smoke-free air.

In the facilitative approach to care the caregiver promotes the right of individuals to make choices, by providing appropriate information to enable effective choices to be made and, where possible, to support the patient to put these choices into action. The difficult obligation that comes with a facilitating approach to care is having the courage to support people to carry their decision-making through, even though this may be accompanied by risks.

People do not choose to be in poverty, or ill or elderly. These are states in which any one of us could find ourselves. At such times our vulnerability should not provide an excuse for others to override our rights. In fact, it could be argued that vulnerability should require that greater efforts are made by others to uphold our rights because the need for protection is greater.

The right to be treated fairly

This right supports the concept that no one should be treated differently from others for irrelevant reasons. In care this can be interpreted as the right to access the same level of care and services as others in similar situations. Being treated fairly does not always mean that individuals should have exactly the same things as other people. The principle of fairness suggests that, where a need is identified, the individual in question is treated no less favourably than those who have a similar need, irrespective of personal attributes. The care that is received should be of the same good standard as that received by others; the quality and competence of the care provided, the time allocated for that care and the attitude in which the care is delivered should not differ. A care practitioner may find it preferable to provide care to someone who is grateful or who is interesting, who is in a particular age group or for whom one has a personal affinity. However, these are irrelevant grounds for distinguishing between people. All people are entitled to the same fair level of care provision irrespective of their attributes.

Right to confidentiality

We have the right to have information about us kept confidential, or to know on what basis information will be shared with others. This subject will be addressed in depth in *Chapter 6*. Therefore, I will only make the point here that confidentiality is, in most cases, a right as long as it does not impinge on the rights or protection of others.

The right to ordinary life opportunities

Being in receipt of care is not an excuse for settling for a second-rate life. The role of welfare provision is to try to ensure service users/patients have access to the same kind of opportunities enjoyed by other members of that community. Therefore, people should have the opportunity to relevant treatments and supportive equipment to enable this to happen. Given that health and social care is funded by a finite resource, the extent of the treatment and support that can be offered is often an issue of conflict and discussion.

The right to competent care provision from service providers

This right means that the people providing care will be more than just 'nice people' although the recent focus on quality of care highlighted in the Francis Report (Francis,

2013) suggests that being nice and in particular caring with kindness are essential criteria for care. Each patient/service user has the right to receive care from someone who has received the appropriate level of training to provide that care. The practitioner has a responsibility to recognise when they have reached the limitations of their knowledge and competence and to know how to access appropriate help or support.

However, competent care is not just about technical ability to perform a skill or activity. Care practitioners have a duty to ensure that their skills are up to date, evidence based, meet latest guidelines and are selected and appropriate for the care they are providing. It is no longer acceptable to continue a practice and justify it on grounds that 'we have always done it this way'. There is now a huge quantity of easily accessible evidence around and practitioners have a duty to try to keep informed about changes in their own field of practice. Equally, employers have an obligation to ensure that opportunities for training and updating are made available to practitioners. Competent care must also be compassionate; patients are not machines to be fixed. Competent care involves kindness, mindfulness and sensitivity to individual vulnerabilities and needs and receptivity to the ways in which the recipient would like their needs to be met.

The right to independent advocacy when requested

At times individuals may not be able to effectively articulate their own needs. In such cases they may need support from someone who can speak on their behalf. Care workers may not be the best people to undertake this role. They may be constrained by professional requirements and obligations to an employer or by a particular point of view. They may also be too closely involved or swayed by their own knowledge and interpretation of the individual's needs and hence be unable to reflect needs accurately. Where users are unable to articulate their own needs they must have the right to access someone who will speak on their behalf.

The right to be accepted for what one is

This right can be seen to embrace the important concepts of equality and anti-discriminatory practice. These rights have been enshrined in law for longer than most other aspects of the Human Rights Act (1998) and they are fundamental to protecting the dignity of minority groups and vulnerable individuals. As such, they warrant some in-depth discussion later in this chapter.

CELEBRATING DIFFERENCE

One of the most prized aspects of human beings is their individuality. No two people are the same. Even identical twins, who share the same genetic code, will display differences in a number of ways. Each one of us wants to be recognised by our own individual identity and personality and to be seen as an independent and worthwhile person in our own right. We seek to illustrate this in the values we adopt, in the activities we engage in and the way we dress (how uncomfortable is it when someone else is wearing the same clothes as you?). The point is that we go to great lengths to make sure that we are different from those around us. When we apply this notion to ourselves in relation to others, difference is good.

ACTIVITY  **4.6**

Think about your friends. Try to identify the ways in which they are all different and what you value about their different attributes.

Hopefully, your friends are not all the same and you value a whole range of attributes in others, you relate to different friends in different ways and for different purposes. For example, you may have one friend who is your confidant, who provides sound advice, or who is just a good listener. However, when you want a friend for a light-hearted fun evening out, you may choose a different friend. These differences do not make either friend less valuable than the other; it is just recognition of difference. These differences are the things that make us interesting. Difference is something to be celebrated.

ACTIVITY **4.7**

Imagine a time when it becomes common practice to treat all people with blonde hair with contempt, either by ignoring them or treating them less well than those with hair of any other colour. This treatment is widely accepted by the rest of society.

- Could this behaviour be rationalised?
- Should I expect everyone with blonde hair to dye it brown in order that they would not be discriminated against?

Given that blonde hair for many people is a matter of genetic lottery, it would seem absurd to suggest that one's worth could be based on such flimsy grounds. However, this is exactly what happens when individuals are discriminated against because of their attributes; those who have a disability, a different race, a particular sexuality or other less tangible characteristics. Individuals may be victimised, ignored or expected to change into something that accords with our beliefs and expectations, rather than being who they are. The thing that makes humans so interesting and so valuable is their difference. We should celebrate it, not penalise people for it.

However, when a difference is something that has not been encountered before, we may feel threatened. Rather than celebrating the difference and trying to see the value of it, we may react negatively. Education in relation to equality and anti-discriminatory practice is designed to help us better understand difference and our reactions to difference, and help us to respect others and value them for what they are.

Equality and anti-discriminatory practice are important considerations in a free and tolerant society that respects and prizes individuality. Likewise, in care practice that supports the notion of the value of the individual, equality and anti-discriminatory practice are important concepts. Both concepts suggest the notion of fairness and justice.

There are numerous policies and legislation in respect of equality and anti-discriminatory practice. Some of the key acts are the Human Rights Act (1998), the Equality Act 2010 (HMSO, 2010) and the Equality and Human Rights Act (2006). This approach to tackling discrimination through law is called the Equal Opportunities Approach (Thompson, 2011). This approach seeks to nullify disadvantage, by ensuring that legal processes protect rights and positively discriminate in favour of disadvantaged, diverse individuals. However, despite this legislation, it remains a fact that inequality and discrimination still persist in health and social care. Policy can only go some of the way to challenge and eradicate discrimination. What is crucially important is how policies are enacted and embedded within day-to-day interactions between practitioners and those in their care. The culture of an organisation plays an important role in how individuals are treated (Tilmouth and Quallington, 2016).

There is a growing recognition that rights are important but not particularly well understood in healthcare. To try to raise awareness and support patient rights, a report and learning programme entitled *Human Rights in Healthcare 2011–12* was published by the government to support practitioners in care environments in upholding others' rights. In addition, *Your Home Care and Human Rights* (Equality and Human Rights Commission, 2012) was published. This guide explains how human rights for those receiving homecare services should be protected.

ACTIVITY 4.8

Read the reports which can be accessed at humanrightsinhealthcare.nhs.uk for examples of good practice in supporting rights.

UNDERSTANDING EQUALITY, PREJUDICE AND DISCRIMINATION

Much of the literature on discrimination and inequality focuses particularly on vulnerable groups; for example, older people, those with disabilities, women, those of different race, people with mental health problems or those of different sexual orientation. It is, of course, important to focus on the specific difficulties faced by individuals in these groups. However, it should not be forgotten that anyone can be discriminated against at any time and the discrimination may have no discernible basis or may be based on a dislike or something equally insubstantial. In addressing issues of equality and discrimination it is necessary to understand what is meant by the terms used.

Equality

Equality does not mean treating everyone the same. Just as people are different, so their needs are different. What is important is that the same principles of fairness are used to establish their need and subsequent treatment. Therefore, equality implies that people should be treated fairly. Applying the principle of equality in practice means that all people in similar situations should be treated similarly. Therefore, all people with a particular type of breast cancer should be offered the same options for treatment. They may not all choose to access the same treatment because their decisions will be based on a range of different personal considerations. However, equality requires that the same opportunities exist for everyone. It is unrealistic to suggest that everyone will be treated exactly the same and situational differences and the dynamics of human interaction make this unlikely, if not impossible. However, there should be no significant differences in treatment offered or behaviours of staff in respect of choices made by patients, unless that difference can be appropriately and convincingly justified.

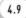 **ACTIVITY** 4.9

Try to think of examples from your own experience of care of people being treated differently even though they had similarities in their needs. For example, two people come into hospital for an identical operation. They have both received preparation and information. One is visibly anxious and has never had surgery before, while the other has had similar operations in the past and is chatting happily with people around her.

Can you suggest reasons for differences in the treatment of individuals and are these reasons persuasive?

You may be looking after two individuals who have had to leave their homes for full-time care in a care home. One of the individuals has made the choice voluntarily and is happy to be there. One has had to reluctantly admit that she can no longer cope and sees the care home as her only option. While it would be very important to help both women settle in well, you may find that you need to adopt very different strategies to do this. Treating people differently may be entirely justifiable as long as the principle of fairness is understood and applied, as a check, and that any material difference can be appropriately explained.

Failure to respect another's right to equality puts them at a disadvantage. Unequal treatment may arise from naivety or the ineffectiveness of the practitioner or because of a pervasive culture which fails to recognise difference. Consider how the needs of a demanding person can take precedence over the needs of someone who sits and waits patiently for their care. Often no malice is intended, and perpetrators may unwittingly trivialise and make a joke of it. However, unfair discrimination is always unacceptable practice and should be guarded against through positive inclusive action (Tilmouth and Quallington, 2016).

Prejudice

Inequality is much more unacceptable when it takes the form of prejudice. Prejudice is an attitude or belief based on a faulty and inflexible generalisation (Thompson, 2011). Discrimination and prejudice are very emotionally loaded words and usually have negative connotations. However, discrimination and prejudice can be positive or favourable in nature. We can hold a particular prejudice that causes us to positively discriminate in favour of someone. There are examples of positive discrimination that help us to combat prejudice; for example the Equality Act (2010) requires organisations to try to recruit a percentage of the workforce with disabilities because, as a group, it is known that they experience significant prejudice and unfair discrimination on irrelevant grounds that have nothing to do with the ability to do the job.

ACTIVITY 4.10

Write down other examples of effective and welcome positive prejudice.

Normally, when we talk about prejudice we are thinking of negative examples of applying 'faulty and negative generalisations'. An example might be the statement 'people are unemployed because they are too lazy to work'. Although this assertion may apply to a small minority, there is substantial evidence to the contrary. It is more widely accepted and demonstrated in research that there are a multitude of complex reasons why someone may be unemployed. Faulty beliefs lead to prejudice. Prejudice can be directed at a group as a whole, or an individual because they are a member of a group. This may be justified by the person holding the prejudice by ascribing particular stereotypical attributes and behaviours to the individual or group who are the focus of the prejudice, as a means of attempting to explain why the prejudice is held. Stereotypical views such as 'women are emotional and illogical' or 'all older adults are hard of hearing' are widely held and believed, even in the face of evidence to the contrary.

How does prejudice manifest itself?

Recent work by Thompson (2011) suggests a prejudice may involve a number of processes:

* **Cognitive** – you develop a false belief that one person or group is better than or superior to another (this belief may develop at a conscious or at an unconscious level; you may, for example, have acquired it from your parents or friends).

- **Emotional** – this belief provokes an emotional response, a feeling towards a particular individual or group that may be dislike or dismissal.
- **Discriminatory action** – this feeling may then be manifested in a number of ways such as, for example, ignoring the person, saying unpleasant things about them to others, deliberately humiliating them or taking some other form of unfair action against them.

Prejudices can be held without resorting to discrimination, and discrimination can occur without prejudice. However, there is frequently a very close and causal link between the two.

Examining prejudice makes individuals feel uncomfortable and most of us would prefer to believe that we do not hold any prejudices. However, it is true to say that we all hold some prejudices. What is important is that we accept that we hold them, we learn to recognise them and we try to eliminate them but, where we cannot, we develop strategies so that they do not lead us into engaging in discriminatory behaviours. Thompson (2006) reminds us that prejudice and subsequent discrimination are rarely confined to the beliefs and actions of an individual but are the result of a combination of influences:

- **Personal beliefs** – those beliefs and values held and acted upon by an individual.
- **Cultural beliefs** – those values held in the social environment that an individual inhabits that strongly influence the individual such as, for example, when, a few years ago, the police service was accused of being 'institutionally racist'.
- **Social and structural beliefs** – these reflect the established social order and are the influence of beliefs, values and divisions in our wider society. There are a number of examples of discriminatory practice of this nature including, for example, the fact that it is only relatively recently (2006) that the law recognised same-sex partnerships.

Sadly, the evidence that inequality and discrimination persist in health and care services is overwhelming.

- An inquiry by Mencap (2012) identified 74 cases of what is claimed to be 'institutional discrimination' in the NHS against those with learning disabilities.
- The report by The King's Fund *Making the Difference: diversity and inclusion in the NHS* (West, Dawson and Kaur, 2015) presents evidence to show that staff who are black, minority and ethnic groups (BME) and other groups such as gay, bisexual, disabled and women are still widely discriminated against in the NHS. If this is how staff are treated, there can be no confidence that patients will be treated any better.
- In 2009 the Department of Health commissioned the Centre for Policy on Ageing to conduct a review of evidence. *Ageism and Age Discrimination in Secondary Health Care in the United Kingdom. A review from the literature* (Centre for Policy on Ageing, 2009) showed that ageism is still a feature of care in the NHS, with

doctors showing slightly more ageist attitudes than other staff. As recently as 2015 there was a flurry of reports in the media claiming ageism in the NHS, with individuals being denied operations and life-saving treatment. The NHS has refuted these claims on the basis that decisions are clinical rather than age related; this is a contentious issue. Whilst much of the evidence needs further study it would suggest that people who work in the NHS treat older people less favourably than they treat other groups.

This evidence of ongoing prejudice and discrimination suggests that care workers are inadequately prepared to work in a non-judgemental and anti-discriminatory manner.

WHY DO DISCRIMINATION AND PREJUDICE CONTINUE TO EXIST IN CARE?

All codes of practice in the fields of health and social care emphasise the need to engage in non-judgemental and anti-discriminatory practice. However, discrimination is still in evidence; there are a number of reasons why this could be so.

- Individuals have a poor or limited understanding of prejudice and anti-discriminatory practice.
- Wherever small groups of workers work in teams there is a tendency to develop particular sets of practices and behaviours. Charles Handy (1997) has likened this to tribes who hold sets of specific and often exclusive tribal behaviours.
- Prejudices, because they can be unconsciously held, can thrive in these environments and might not be recognised as people become immune due to constant exposure. New staff to an area may initially be aware of prejudicial practices but, as they become part of the everyday experience (as long as the practices are not extreme), the new staff member may quickly adapt to the behaviours themselves in an effort to belong to the existing group, and so the behaviours are perpetuated.
- There are organisational policies or constraints which support discriminatory practice.
- The power imbalance between the carer and the cared-for supports an environment in which the individual in receipt of care will always be at risk of anti-discriminatory behaviour.
- Likes and dislikes of individuals or groups can result in discrimination.
- Care practitioners may believe that individuals who are different should, as far as possible, conform to the majority or less different position.

ACTIVITY 4.11

How valid do you think these explanations are? Can you suggest any other explanations for why discrimination continues to exist?

ENGAGING IN ANTI-DISCRIMINATORY PRACTICE

Treating service users and carers fairly is one of the core duties of a care practitioner. Unfair treatment increases vulnerability and causes disadvantage. There are a number of principles that emerge from literature regarding how inequality and discrimination can be tackled in practice. Twelvetrees (2002) suggests three ways of tackling inequality by changing our approach:

- celebrate diversity – 'reframe difference' so that sharing different views and accepting varied choices are positive activities that enhance our knowledge and experience
- challenge oppression – when we see oppression from others we question and challenge it, or refuse to be part of it
- empower the oppressed – power or perceived power is often exercised by those who engage in discrimination so, if we can help to empower those who are seen as vulnerable, we can help break the cycle of discrimination.

How can these principles be applied to a care environment?

Celebrate diversity

Even if you work with one service user group think about the things that make each individual different. Even when you do not particularly like someone it is usually possible to find a redeeming feature or some attribute that you admire, so focus on the positive not the negative.

Challenge oppression

When people talk in denigrating ways about others we should question it and refuse to engage with jokes that reinforce stereotypes and prejudice. Ask questions about why certain practices are followed, as this may bring hitherto unrecognised issues into the open. There is no need to be directly confrontational; merely not engaging in the practice or questioning something stops the reinforcement of it.

Empower the oppressed

In recent years the introduction of advocacy schemes and user and carer involvement initiatives have gone some way to empowering others. However, empowerment need not be at this formal level but can be as simple as establishing a relationship of equality and respect with the individual in your care and taking time to listen to and, where possible, action their views and needs.

Recognising prejudice

It is essential to reflect on your own possible prejudices. We cannot begin to combat something if we do not acknowledge that it exists. Ask yourself questions such as: 'what prejudices do I hold?' and 'where do they come from and why?' Challenge your prejudices. Examine your care practice. Did you spend more time or better quality time with one person in your care rather than another person? Why is this? Is there any evidence that could be based on prejudice? What strategies could you use to overcome your prejudices?

ACTIVITY 4.12

Reflect on the organisation and context in which you deliver care. Does your organisation unwittingly reinforce discrimination or support anti-discriminatory practice?

These are examples of how you can begin to think about anti-discriminatory practice and question practice:

- Are there any policies or practices that discriminate against individuals on the basis of age or other irrelevant criteria?
- Do you have any practices that favour opportunities for one service user over another?
- Are there any areas that are inaccessible to some service users because of their disabilities?
- Do you provide interpretation for those whose first language is not English?
- Do you hold service user meetings at a time or venue that is difficult for those with disabilities or carers to attend?
- Do you have a philosophy in the organisation that promotes empowerment?

Inequality often results from thoughtlessness and insensitivity rather than from any premeditated desire to hurt or disenfranchise others. It is the responsibility of the healthcare practitioner to be reflective of their own attitudes and behaviours to ensure that they are alert to possible discriminatory practice.

CASE STUDY 4.1

Mrs Kowalski is a Jewish lady of Polish origin who has just started coming to the day centre in which you work. When you come on duty you are told that she is introverted and difficult. She has not eaten or drunk anything that has been given to her, she refuses to join in the activities that are put on and seems reluctant to answer questions. She has been incontinent twice and staff are considering whether she is a suitable candidate for this service, which would be better going to someone else who would appreciate it. You notice that staff are avoiding contact with her. This is the first time that Mrs Kowalski has been in a care environment. She does not speak English well and has difficulty hearing people because of her deteriorating hearing. She has been an orthodox Jew all her life and only eats kosher food.

- Which of Mrs Kowalaski's rights are not being met?
- What could you do in order to improve her experience of care?

A RIGHTS-BASED APPROACH TO CARE

It may have become obvious that a rights-focused approach to care is aimed at protecting and furthering the independence and opportunities of all individuals. Rights are a particularly useful tool for vulnerable people to use to challenge unfair treatment, inequality and discrimination. However, rights cannot be easily separated from responsibilities. In the discussion about rights far less attention has been paid to the corresponding responsibilities that go hand in hand with rights. It needs to be recognised that to be in legitimate receipt of rights, someone has a responsibility to provide for that right and that individual will action that agreement. If they fail in this duty, in relation to an explicit right, there is a case to answer. However, the recipient of rights might also have responsibilities. If I want to exercise the right to have my individual needs met I must accept the responsibility to try to articulate effectively what those needs are; it is unreasonable to expect another to guess what those specific needs might be. I may also be responsible for working in partnership with the care practitioner to ensure that the rights are met.

CONCLUSION

A rights-based approach to care is based upon the core values of care and rights are claimed against those core values. Rights are entitlements and protections and claims against them are often made when individuals feel that their rights are not being met or that they are being treated unfairly. The problem in asserting rights and claims is that it can be confrontational and adversarial. It can be argued that a rights-based society can lead to a society in which individuals selfishly care more about the fulfilment of their individual rights than they do about the state of society as a whole, or about individuals who are in a worse situation than themselves. An alternative approach is for society to strive to identify the rights and respect that all citizens should enjoy and ensure that this respect and these rights are afforded to all, without an individual having to fight for them. However, this discussion is beyond the scope of this chapter.

CHAPTER SUMMARY

Seven key points to take away from Chapter 4:

- Rights are an important feature of care in western societies.
- There are many different kinds of rights.
- Rights are often resorted to when individuals feel they are not receiving what they are entitled to.
- Rights provide a vehicle for people to articulate their needs.
- Rights cannot be separated from responsibilities.
- Discriminatory practices still occur in care practice.
- Practitioners need to reflect on their practice and develop strategies to eliminate unfair discrimination.

FURTHER READING

Bateman, N. (2006) *Practising Welfare Rights*. Abingdon: Routledge.

Centre for Policy on Ageing (2009) *Ageism and Age Discrimination in Secondary Health Care in the United Kingdom*. London: CPA.

Equality and Human Rights Commission website: www.equalityhumanrights.com

Human Rights in Health Care website: humanrightsinhealthcare.nhs.uk/About-Us/human_rights_in_healthcareprot_ld.aspx

Thompson, N. (2011) *Promoting Equality: working with diversity and difference*. Basingstoke: Palgrave Macmillan.

Tilmouth, T. and Quallington, J. (2016) Chapter 5 in *Level 5 Diploma in Leadership for Health and Social Care*. 2nd ed. London: Hodder Education.

05

RESPECT AND DIGNITY

LEARNING OUTCOMES:

In this chapter you will:

- define respect and dignity and consider what it means to be respectful and to have respect for others

- identify the moral justification for a duty of respect for persons and consider the notion of personhood

- discuss duties and rules arising from the value of respect for persons and their implications for practice

- explore the concepts of dignity and privacy in relation to practice

- reflect on care strategies that promote respect and dignity.

INTRODUCTION

People value their dignity. While they may not identify exactly what this means, they know when it has been compromised or threatened. People are particularly vulnerable to loss of dignity in healthcare as their care needs bring what is normally private into the public realm and require the intervention of relative strangers. Dignity is closely associated with the values of respect (of self and others), respect for persons and respect for a person's autonomy. We will discuss autonomy in detail in *Chapter 6*.

Recognition of your humanity through respect for you as a person is fundamental to maintaining your dignity and to your feelings of self-esteem and self-worth. These notions of respect and dignity have attracted considerable attention in recent years, both in theory and in practice. They are at the forefront of government policy and are reflected in a range of government reports, particularly in responses to inquiries into incidents of poor and inhumane care (DH, 2014; 2012; 2012a and b; DH and Poulter, 2013; Francis, 2013).

Professional and policy expectations of respect and dignity

Respecting people and their dignity are fundamental expectations for you as a practitioner and core values for all health and care services, reflected in national standards and strategies throughout the UK.

Respect and dignity are:
- principal values in the NHS Constitution (DH, 2015a, p.5)
- central to the vision and strategy for nursing, midwifery and care staff (DH and NHS Commissioning Board, 2012c)
- fundamental aspects of care in the *Essence of Care 2010* benchmark (DH, 2010b)
- central to the mental health strategy, *No Health without Mental Health* (DH, 2011a)
- featured in the fundamental standards in 'The Health and Social Care Act 2008 (Regulated Activities) Regulations 2014' (DH, 2014a, b, and c)
- key values in the National Occupational Standards for Health and Social Care (2013) (see *Box 5.1*)
- integral to the *Core Competences for Healthcare Support Workers and Adult Social Care Workers in England* (Skills for Care and Skills for Health, 2013b)
- reinforced in the *Care Certificate Standards* for healthcare support workers (HCSW) and adult social care workers (ASCW) (Health Education England, Skills for Care and Skills for Health, 2015).

BOX 5.1

The National Occupational Standards for Health and Social Care (2013)

These identify the principles and values that underpin the rights that individuals (children, young people and adults) and key people have:

- to be treated as an individual
- to be treated equally and not be discriminated against
- to be respected
- to have privacy
- to be treated in a dignified way
- to be protected from danger and harm
- to be supported and cared for in a way that meets their needs, takes account of their choices and also protects them
- to communicate using their preferred methods of communication and language
- to access information about themselves.

See for example: National Occupational Standard (SCDHSC0234) *Uphold the Rights of Individuals* (Skills for Care and Development, March 2012) available at tools.skillsforhealth.org.uk/external/SCDHSC0234.pdf (accessed 14 December 2016)

Health and social care professions view respect as fundamental to the healthcare relationship, both with patients, service users and their families as well as respecting each other as members of the care team. Respecting 'dignity, humanity and equality' is one of the key *Principles of Nursing Practice* identified by the Royal College of Nursing (RCN) (Jackson and Irwin, 2011). Similarly, Skills for Care identify seven core principles essential to supporting dignity in adult social care (Skills for Care, 2013).

The concepts of respect, individual autonomy and preservation of dignity are also fundamental to many codes of practice and professional conduct for health and care practitioners such as the *Code of Conduct for Healthcare Support Workers and Adult Social Care Workers in England* (Skills for Care and Skills for Health, 2013a) and the *Standards of Proficiency for Social Workers in England* (Health and Care Professions Council, 2017).

The Code: professional standards of practice and behaviour for nurses and midwives (NMC, 2015) puts 'prioritising the interests of people' first. This expects practitioners to treat people as individuals and uphold their dignity, listen and respond to people's preferences and concerns, make sure that people's physical, social and psychological needs are assessed and responded to, act in the best interests of people at all times and respect people's right to privacy and confidentiality (NMC, 2015, pp.2–6).

The right to be treated with respect and dignity is also enshrined in law, with various pieces of legislation supporting this legal right, most significantly the Human Rights Act (1998) and the Equality Act (2010) but also laws associated with mental capacity, data protection and freedom of information.

Despite all this, incidents of poor care continue, and certain groups of patients and service users have been particularly vulnerable to disrespect and undignified care resulting in significant harms and loss of self-worth and self-esteem. These include older people, people with learning disabilities, and those with dementia or mental health problems. For example, the National Service Framework (NSF) for Older People (DH, 2001a) aimed to address the widespread infringement of dignity of older people. Yet respect and dignity were still found lacking in the care of older people a decade later (Parliamentary and Health Service Ombudsman, 2011).

Similarly, *Valuing People: a new strategy for learning disability for the 21st century* (DH, 2001b) emphasised the importance of placing the individual with learning disabilities at the centre of care. But respect, dignity and person-centred care and support for people with learning disabilities, their families and carers were still found wanting and their importance re-emphasised in *Valuing People Now* (DH, 2009) and *Transforming Care: a national response to Winterbourne View Hospital* (DH, 2012b). However, the values of respect for persons and dignity are not exclusive to particular service user groups. They are relevant to whoever you will meet in your practice, including staff and other carers, and in your everyday life.

Despite many references to the values of respect and dignity in health and social care policy, codes and guidelines, assumptions are made about practitioners sharing a common understanding of these concepts. As dilemmas in care indicate, these values are more complex in their meaning and their application than professional rules for practice alone can convey.

This chapter aims to develop a deeper understanding of the moral values of respect for persons, dignity and privacy and explores their centrality to good health and social care. It encourages reflection on the attitudes and behaviours that impact on an individual's dignity and sense of self-worth and supports development of care strategies that promote respect for persons and dignity-enhancing care.

WHAT DO WE MEAN WHEN WE USE THE TERMS 'RESPECT' AND 'RESPECT FOR PERSONS'?

Thinking about respect as a value

Respect is important to daily life, although this is often equated with simply respecting the authority of others, such as people in power, the law or religion. The word 'respect' has become commonplace in everyday language, both in the general public domain (for example, respecting nature and the environment, respect for human life in debates about abortion, respecting cultural difference and diversity) and in political debate. For example, the UK coalition government of 2010–15 espoused a commitment to building a fairer society and to support social action to change culture and attitudes through the 'Equality Strategy', with the aim of 'building respect for all, tackling discrimination, hate crime and violence' (HM Government, 2010).

Respect for self and others is a fundamental element of living together in a society. However, there are many ways to think about and use the term 'respect' and it may have different meanings to different people and according to the context in which it is used, such as 'respect me for who I am' or 'respect my authority'. Both of these demand acknowledgement, recognition and consideration by others, although the reason for giving (or owing) such respect is different.

ACTIVITY 5.1

Reflection

Have you ever experienced a time when you felt that you were not respected or felt undervalued? This may have been, for example, in a family or personal relationship, in an interaction with someone you know or with a stranger, or in a work environment.

- Describe this significant incident. Where were you? Who was involved? Were there any specific circumstances?
- Then think about and write down:
  - How did this make you feel?
  - Why did you feel this way?
  - What did you do?

You may have identified a number of feelings, such as anger, upset, sadness, disbelief, concern, being belittled. It may have been harder to identify exactly why you felt this way; you may have felt that it just wasn't 'fair' or 'right'. However, it is important as a reflective practitioner that you keep asking yourself why you believe something is right or wrong or should or should not be the way it is. You may have said that it was disrespectful of you as an individual. This idea of respect and respect for persons needs further exploration.

Defining respect

There are various ways to define respect. The term 'respect' can refer simply to a *behaviour* that avoids violating or interfering with a boundary or rule; for example, a driver respecting a speed limit or a smoker refraining from smoking in public places. Respect can also involve an *attitude or feeling*, as when we speak of having respect for another person. Practitioners in health and care are expected to respect boundaries or rules, such as the law associated with consent to treatment, policies, competencies for practice and the rules outlined in codes of conduct. However, what we are most concerned about here are the *values and attitudes* associated with 'respect for persons' and their influence on a practitioner's behaviours and practice.

ACTIVITY 5.2

Defining respect

1. Think about and write down your definition of 'respect'.

2. If you find this difficult, start a concept map showing different words, phrases and ideas that come to mind when you think about 'respect' (you may well identify many more words and ideas than indicated by the six arrows below).

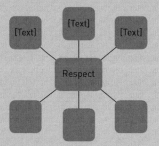

3. Look up 'respect' in a dictionary and add the definition to your 'mind map' (but remember a dictionary definition will only start to identify its meaning).

4. Now talk to some relatives, friends and/or colleagues about their understanding of the term 'respect'.

5. Try rewriting your definition now.

Respect in the health and care context can be simply defined as the recognition of the *unconditional value of patients, service users, clients and carers as persons*. This requires both *a belief* that persons should be valued and that your *actions should reflect such a belief* (Beach *et al.*, 2007). Respect seen in this way necessarily involves respecting autonomy but this alone is not a sufficient understanding of respect for persons in care relationships. Respect can mean not only a symbolic recognition of status or social position but also paying proper attention to the 'object' of respect and acknowledgement of the value and worth of something or someone. Thus, being respectful reflects an individual's:

- beliefs
- evaluative judgements
- commitments
- dispositions of attitude and behaviour towards the person who is being respected.

ACTIVITY 5.3

Reflection

- Think of a situation where you feel that another person has been treated with disrespect. Identify what form/s of respect were disregarded. Was it someone's authority or position that was ignored or undermined? Was it the attitude of a person towards another that seemed disrespectful? Were any rules or boundaries broken? Was it a combination of some or all of these factors?
- Can you identify why the person was treated this way?
- In your view, how should this situation have been handled? What should have happened?

The principle of respect for persons

As children we are generally taught to respect significant others such as parents, elders, teachers and people 'in authority'. As we get older, we may develop a deeper understanding of respectfulness and the value of respect for others, connected with their feelings, rights and differing opinions. We may have great respect for some people based purely on a positive assessment of their merits or social standing and consider them exemplary; we may lose respect for others, depending on our judgement of whether they are truly worthy of our respect. We may also come to believe that all people are worthy of respect, regardless of whether they display any merits, because of their humanity, as unique individuals and simply because they are persons.

Respect for persons as persons should be distinguished from respect for persons in particular roles or based only on the positive assessment of the merits of an individual. Respect for persons is not simply about 'liking' or even 'agreeing with' someone. Although it involves an emotional response, it is not merely about sentiment but requires a corresponding disposition to respond and act respectfully towards the 'object' of respect, the person. Equally, respect is more than just respectful behaviour, because simply to behave in a way that appears respectful, without valuing that respect, is deceitful. The idea of paying proper attention to the person central to your respect means trying to see the person clearly in their own right and through their own eyes; trying to identify their values, desires, strengths, wants and needs and not seeing them solely through the filter of your own feelings and dispositions (Dillon, 2014).

The *motive* behind your show of respect for another person is as morally important as knowing how to act respectfully. For example, not using racially inappropriate language while caring for an Asian family simply because you do not want to be caught breaching race discrimination laws is not sufficient motive to be considered respectful. In this case, your fear of legal recrimination is more about self-interest than the value of respect for others, even though on one level you are showing respect for the authority of the law. The motive for your action should come from the value you attributed to them as persons with equal rights to respect and because you believe all individuals are unique and valued members of society.

Dillon (2014) identifies what he calls 'care respect', which

'... involves regarding the object [of respect] as having profound and perhaps unique value and so cherishing it, and perceiving it as fragile or calling for special care and so acting or forbearing to act out of felt benevolent concern for it.'

(Dillon, 2014, p.7, Sect. 1.2)

Thinking of respect as 'care respect' encompasses the belief that persons have a unique value deserving of special concern and care.

Harris (1985, p.193) adds, 'having concern for the welfare of others' as another essential component of respect for persons. Concern for the welfare of others may be mutually compatible with respect for autonomy (often associated with respect for persons), although many moral dilemmas in health and social care practice arise when these two values come into conflict, as you will see when we talk about risk, protection from harms and acting in a person's best interests.

BOX 5.2

Respect for persons

This at the very least requires:

- a belief in the value of persons as individuals and as members of society
- an obligation to respect individuals as human beings
- treating people in the manner in which you would expect to be treated
- showing consideration for another person's feelings and interests
- an attitude demonstrating that you value another person.

Many of the ordinary rules and judgements of common social morality (our ordinary shared moral beliefs) presuppose respect for persons as a foundation of all other moral principles, duties and obligations. In this way, the principle of respect for persons can be considered to be *universal* and should not have any national, cultural, legal, or economic boundaries. This is evident in much of the discussion of values and ethics associated with health and social care, where respect for persons and the worth of all human beings is seen as an essential guiding principle that underpins all others (Banks, 2012; Beauchamp and Childress, 2013; Seedhouse, 2009). For example, if you act according to the principle that it is wrong to harm another then this will, in part, be based in you valuing their humanity and them as a unique individual, with feelings and interests that should not be violated.

THE MORAL DUTY OF RESPECT FOR PERSONS

Much of the contemporary discussion of respect for persons is credited to the work of an eighteenth-century German philosopher, Immanuel Kant, who put respect for persons at the very centre of his deontological moral theory. His original writings are complex and open to misinterpretation but some of the key points from his work are relevant to the value of respect for persons in care practice.

Kant argued that all people are bearers of fundamental rights and that persons have an absolute dignity that is independent of rank or merit and must always be respected. Thus, persons have absolute value, unconditional worth and exist as 'ends in themselves', in contrast to things that are valuable merely as a means to an end or as objects of affection. This value is common to all people and is concerned not with being human beings in a genetic sense, but with our humanity and the associated possession of the special features that make us *distinctively human*. This includes the capacities of 'reason and freedom of will', i.e. the ability for self-directed rational behaviour and to choose and follow our own moral goals. We will come back to some of these ideas in the discussion of respect for autonomy in *Chapter 6*.

Kant stated his principle of respect for persons as a 'categorical imperative'; an absolute requirement that *we should always act in ways that treat humanity as an end in itself, never merely or exclusively as a means to another person's ends*.

Thinking about this statement, you should be able to recognise that there is something intuitively wrong in treating human beings as merely instruments to achieve our own goals. An extreme example of this would be slavery. However, this does not totally rule out using people for our own purposes and we do this on a regular basis. For example, when I employ a plumber to fix my central heating, I am using him as a means to my own ends. What is important, however, is that I am not treating him *merely* as a means to my own ends because, in employing him, we both enter freely into a 'contract' (in this instance, involving payment). The plumber is able to make choices as to whether or not he wants to do this work or something else, he can influence when he is available, how much it will cost, etc. The same can be said of any person employed to provide a service, paid or voluntary, including care workers, as they have all chosen to enter into their role and with some purpose of their own. Conversely, a slave is treated as a means to someone else's ends, they are not free to make choices about how they live their life and their sole purpose is to fulfil another person's wishes and commands.

One example of the notion of 'using people as a means to an end' in healthcare occurs when human research subjects are recruited to participate in trials for the testing of a new drug or treatment, as they are obviously being used for the potential benefit of others. Some people may get involved for *altruistic reasons*; their contribution to improving treatments for others and society. Others will do it for *their own benefits*, including financial reward, or they may have both motives. In either case, they have not been used merely as a means to another's ends; they also had a purpose to their involvement and a choice to participate or not. This is morally permissible, provided they made their decision freely and that the necessary conditions for informed choice and consent have been met, such as the provision of sound information. These expectations for consent relate closely to the principle of respect for autonomy to be discussed in *Chapter 6*. There are rigorous guidelines for the ethical approval and conduct of medical research, which up to 2016 included the Research Governance Framework for Health and Social Care (DH, 2005b). The Health Research Authority (HRA) will publish a new UK policy framework for health and social care research following consultation in 2016 (HRA, 2016). However, the application of published rules and guidelines still depends on the moral integrity and values of the people conducting and participating in research and on those that make judgements on the nature and moral imperative of the research itself in approving the research proposal.

Due respect for humanity

What Kant also required was not just a sense of respect for others but that, morally speaking, you should act with *due respect for humanity*. On this basis, you should foster an attitude of due respect rather than simply a 'feeling' of respect. This is particularly pertinent to a value-based approach to caring for others. We owe persons respect simply because *they are persons*, regardless of whether we like them, they are useful to us or even if they have wronged us. Think about the value of respect for persons as you consider *Case study 5.1*.

Alfred in A & E

Gemma is a healthcare assistant. She usually works in a medical ward but she has been sent to cover the evening shift in Accident and Emergency. Alfred, an elderly man, is brought in by ambulance; he is unkempt and smells strongly of alcohol. His clothes are stained with urine. He is well-known to the locals; he is homeless and has been living on the streets for several years. Some passers-by called the ambulance when they saw him fall down a small flight of steps. Following initial assessment, he has no serious injuries but he has grazes on his hands and a small cut on his forehead. He is to be kept in overnight for observation. Staff usually take this opportunity to provide basic hygiene and clean clothes. Gemma is asked to wash Alfred's hands and face and to stay with him until a registered nurse is available to suture the cut. However, he has become extremely vocal, is swearing at any member of staff that goes near him and he is disturbing other patients and relatives. As she enters the cubicle, Alfred hurls verbal abuse at her and, when she offers to wash the blood from his hands and face and to get him some clean clothes, Alfred pushes her away forcefully.

Gemma starts to think that she's drawn the short straw. She doesn't see why she should subject herself to Alfred's vile language and abuse and if that's the way he feels and he doesn't want helping, then why should she bother? It is Alfred's choice after all.

- What are your initial feelings about this case? Should Alfred's desire to be left alone be respected? Provide a justification for your answer.
- Can a person forfeit their right to be respected? If so, give some examples of your reasoning.

This is an example where the desire to provide care and act in what you believe to be a person's best interests can come into conflict with duties arising from respect for them as persons, a conflict made more complex in this case by the individual's behaviour. You may feel that Alfred's behaviour is unacceptable and there are limits to what you should have to endure in providing care, as you too are deserving of respect as an individual. However, in these kinds of situations, it is not the case that the patient no longer deserves respect for their humanity or as a person, even if they have quite different interpretations from yours of what is in their best interests. You may have identified that Gemma had obligations to ensure (as far as possible) Alfred's safety while in hospital, although this does not extend to insisting that he washes and changes his clothing.

Tadd *et al.*'s (2011) research of older people in acute hospital settings identified issues associated with risk management and the 'unintended consequences' for a person's self-respect and dignity. The priority given to safety and risk management is often appropriate and both patients and their relatives have interests in being kept safe and to prevent them coming to harm (we explore this further in *Chapter 8*). However, they concluded that attempts to minimise uncertainties through clinical governance and the regulation of risk can impact on approaches to care delivery as staff become unduly risk-averse. Such approaches then threaten respect for individuals and their dignity.

Tadd *et al.* (2011, pp.90–91) describe practice where concerns for patient safety, particularly for confused patients or those with dementia, meant that staff focused much of their time in preventing patients from moving out of their chairs. They found other examples where patients' freedom and mobility were restricted, such as the use of bed rails, being told to stay sitting down, or being placed in a wheelchair, thus preventing their ability to stand. Care practices tended to be risk averse and did not balance the risk of falling with the possibilities of harm to the person's sense of worth, their identity and their dignity.

Tadd *et al.*'s (2011) work formed part of the Prevention of Abuse and Neglect in the Institutional Care of Older Adults (PANICOA) research initiative. The studies drew on the priorities of older people, their relatives and carers and the summary report identifies eight core 'domains' of the overall care experience that would benefit from improvement in policy and practice, including 'dignity and respect', 'involvement and control', 'communication and information', 'community and relationships' and 'identity and meaning'. These informed two 'Templates for Good Practice', which include specific actions necessary to ensure a 'respect and protect' care culture (Lupton and Croft-White, 2013, pp.4–5).

You may also have considered in *Case study 5.1* whether Alfred was capable of understanding what was in his best interests at this time and whether he was in full control of his decision-making and behaviour, particularly if he was under the influence of alcohol. This links to the discussion of competence and capacity in personal autonomy in *Chapter 6*, but may also raise questions of how we define 'persons' when we talk about the value of respect for persons and those deserving of respect.

Defining the 'person'

One consideration important to the discussion of respect for persons is whether the terms 'human being' and 'person' are synonymous. There are two common interpretations of the term 'human being'. First, a human being is a member of the species *Homo sapiens*; this has genetic, biological and scientific relevance. However, when we refer to the value of human life we mean much more than a preference for our own species. What is often intended when we talk about the value of the 'human being' is consideration of what makes them a 'person'.

Recognition as a 'person' is significant in society because it lies at the centre of debates about the status, respect, rights and treatments that are obligatory to different types of living beings. Thus, the value of respect for persons inevitably requires some definition of what is meant by 'persons' although this in itself can be contentious. For example, in philosophy and applied ethics, the definition of 'person' used can often exclude human beings who are incapable of certain kinds of thought, such as embryos, fetuses, newborn infants or adult humans who lack the capacity for higher brain functions. There are many definitions of 'person' put forward in the literature that incorporate a wide range of defining characteristics and the recognition of status as a person is known as 'personhood'.

One significant definition of 'persons' comes again from Kant who makes assumptions about 'persons' being rational beings, capable of self-determination, where rationality relates to being able to give reasons for your actions and self-determination means being able to make decisions and act according to your own choices and desires (Banks, 2012, p.43). Kant also saw persons as having the ability to determine their own moral rules and obligations that guide their actions, and that it is this that makes them intrinsically valuable.

Other common characteristics that feature in definitions of the 'person' include:
- possessing human genetic material
- having potential for human development
- the necessity of birth
- personal identity
- individuality
- presence of self-concept and self-awareness
- a sense of self that persists through time
- someone capable of valuing their own existence
- development of communication and language
- the ability to reason
- reflective capacity.

Further definitions of persons and personhood can be seen in *Box 5.3*.

If you hold the view that persons are identified simply by 'being human', i.e. the possession of human genetic material, then this would suggest that some of the practices that society already endorses are -immoral, for example, termination of pregnancy (which does concur with some people's views). However, you can see in the definitions in *Box 5.3*, that persons can be defined as beings capable of having interests that other living things do not, or cannot, have and suggests that it is these capacities that lead us to attribute value to persons.

If you believe the value of people is based purely in their capacity to be rational, self-determining, able to value themselves and to reason, then there could be a significant number of people to whom any duty of respect would not be owed, such as those with complex learning disabilities, severe mental health problems or some forms of dementia. To judge who is owed respect simply on the basis of such capacities does not sit well with our intuitions about valuing and respecting humanity. Also, there

Some definitions of persons and personhood

Singer (1993, p.86) refers to Fletcher's (1972) 'indicators of humanhood', seeing these to be synonymous with personhood, i.e:

- self-awareness
- self-control
- a sense of the future
- a sense of the past
- the capacity to relate to others
- concern for others
- communication
- curiosity.

Locke (1690, cited by Gillon, 1986, p.51) defined a 'person' as

'... a thinking intelligent being that has reason and reflection and can consider itself as itself, the same thinking being in different times and place; which is inseparable from thinking and as it seems to me essential to it.'

Warren (1973) includes in her definition of the 'person' possession of:

- consciousness... (particularly) the capacity to feel pain
- reasoning (the developed capacity to solve new and relatively complex problems)
- self-motivated activity
- the capacity to communicate... on indefinitely many possible topics
- the presence of self-concepts, and self-awareness.

According to Lockwood (1985, p.10), a person

'... must have the capacity for reflective consciousness and self-consciousness. It must have, or at any rate have the ability to acquire, a concept of itself, as a being with a past and a future.'

may be many beings who are not rational and self-conscious (thus not fulfilling these criteria of personhood) and yet are capable of experiencing pleasure and suffering and to whom we would still attribute value and respect. Singer (1993, p.101) refers to these as *conscious beings*. Many non-human animals may well fall into this category but it could also include, for example, newborn infants and those in persistent vegetative states.

People may also retain the ability to value one thing over another and exhibit this through emotional and non-verbal responses even after they have lost the rational ability to formulate and communicate a particular decision, as with severe dementia. These abilities

Persons worthy of respect?

- Can you identify any potential problems in your practice if the definitions of persons identified in *Box 5.3* were to be used in judgements of who (or what kinds of people) should be worthy of respect?

- Make a list of examples where there may be conflict with the above definitions of persons.

- Talk to friends or colleagues about what features in your list. Do they agree? If not, what are the reasons for their differences of opinion?

- For example, these definitions are commonly used as just one of the arguments to justify the act of abortion, i.e. if the fetus is not capable of reasoning and self-awareness then it is not a person. It then follows, in this argument, that if the fetus is not a person, it is not deserving of the same level of respect as the 'fully fledged' human being. Therefore, on this account, termination of pregnancy is morally permissible.

to value may still be evident through gestures and emotions, for example, to music or pets (Nuffield Council on Bioethics, 2009). Thus, valuing conscious life and the very fact that someone *is human* is as important as valuing 'personhood' as defined by rationality, and emphasises that respect and dignity relate to every human regardless of their capacities; hence why we have talked here about respect for humanity as well as persons.

It is the commonly held notions of personhood that include rationality and their interpretation, which can cause dilemmas in practice, including in judgements about an individual's competence and capacity to be autonomous in their decisions about their own care. Such dilemmas can give rise to paternalism, where a person's own autonomous choices or preferences are overridden on the grounds that you believe you are acting in their best interests, although paternalism is sometimes too easily dismissed and confused with motives of exploitation and control. We explore paternalism further in *Chapter 6*.

Challenging the classic rationality-based view of personhood

Tom Kitwood's (1997) work on dementia and person-centred care challenged the classic rationality and capacity-based view of personhood. He argued for the recognition of *the person* in every individual, regardless of how advanced their dementia was. He claimed that despite loss of function and capacity, persons with dementia do not lose their essential *non-cognitive attributes of humanity*. Thus, even if the person's mood, behaviour and memory change quite profoundly, the person with severe dementia is still the same *person* as before the onset of dementia. Other factors support their identity as a person, such as their physical presence and their interpersonal identity established through relationships with others. Kitwood (1993) viewed agency, sociability and sentience (the ability to feel, perceive, or experience) as the central attributes of persons and described personhood as:

> '... a status or standing bestowed upon one human being, by others, in the context of social relationship and social being. It implies recognition, respect and trust.'
>
> (Kitwood, 1997, p.8)

Thus, although carers and relatives may refer to someone with dementia as not being 'the same person' as they once were, this tends not to be meant literally but due to changes in behaviour and mood which can be distressing and generate feelings of loss (Nuffield Council on Bioethics, 2009).

In addition, Kitwood viewed personhood as transcendent, sacred, and unique, affording absolute value to people with dementia and resulting in an obligation, '... to treat each other with deep respect.' (Kitwood, 1997, p.8).

In establishing his philosophy of person-centred care, Kitwood demonstrated how personhood could be eroded by the actions of carers, even if these were not maliciously intended. He termed the adverse effects of these actions on the wellbeing of people with dementia, 'Malignant Social Psychology' (Innes, 2009). These interactions, what he called 'Personal Detractions', could range from mild (when no malice was intended) through to very severe (when a carer was aware of the impact their actions would have on the person with dementia). Kitwood identified seventeen 'personal detractions' which are incompatible with respect for persons and potentially damaging to a person's dignity regardless of whether they have dementia (Kitwood, 1997, pp.46–7):

- Treachery
- Disempowerment
- Infantilisation
- Intimidation
- Labelling
- Stigmatisation
- Outpacing
- Invalidation
- Banishment
- Objectification
- Ignoring
- Imposition
- Withholding
- Accusation
- Disruption
- Mockery
- Disparagement.

You may well recognise some of these approaches from your experiences of care practice or in your everyday life. They need not be stark, malicious approaches but could be quite subtle interactions, for example 'talking over' an individual and asking a relative for information about medications without involving the person concerned. Think back to *Activity 3.1* in Chapter 3. The nurse involved was at least guilty of ignoring what she was told about the woman's discomfort, which led to disempowerment and infantilisation, and some degree of objectification through concentrating on the medical aspects of the woman's treatment rather than her 'holistic care', comfort and wellbeing.

Kitwood (1997) claimed that the personhood of individuals with dementia could be maintained through *person-centred care*. He placed the individual at the very centre of dementia care through creating and sustaining meaningful relationships with, and genuine concern for, the individual. Although Kitwood's account is not without criticism (for example, Nolan *et al.*, 2002), Dewing (2008) reminds us that Kitwood's ultimate purpose was of that of the *moral concern for 'others'*. This accords with respect for humanity and with the accounts of compassion previously explored.

Building on Kitwood's vision of care, Brooker (2003, 2007) identified four major elements (VIPS) that define her concept of person-centred care and Brooker and Latham (2015) use the 'VIPS framework' to promote service improvement through person-centred dementia care. The VIPS elements are (Brooker and Latham, 2015, pp.12–13):
- *Valuing people* with dementia and those who care for them; promoting their rights and entitlements regardless of age or cognitive impairment (V)
- Treating people as *individuals*; appreciating that all people with dementia have a unique history, identity, personality and physical, psychological, social and economic resources, and that these will affect their response to cognitive impairments (I)
- Viewing the world from the *perspective of the person* with dementia; recognising that each person's experience has its own psychological validity (P)
- Recognising that all human life, including that of people with dementia, is grounded in relationships and that people with dementia need an enriched *social environment* that compensates for their impairment and fosters opportunity for personal growth and relative wellbeing (S).

You should be able to see similarities between these elements of person-centred dementia care and the values of compassion and care identified earlier and the notion of social-relational autonomy in *Chapter 6*.

Although defining persons is not straightforward, the value of 'respect for persons' is a starting point for good morality because it accepts the basic premise that other people matter, and this is an important value in a societal context. Humans do not live as isolated beings and, consequently, mutual respect should be a fundamental principle. Downie and Telfer (1969) characterise respect as 'valuing and cherishing

ACTIVITY 5.5

Using the VIPS elements to guide reflection on your interactions with people with dementia and their families (adapted from Brooker, 2012), ask yourself:

- Does my behaviour and the manner in which I am communicating with this person show that I respect, value and honour them?

- Am I treating this person as a unique individual with a history and a wide range of strengths and needs?

- Am I making a serious attempt to see my actions from the perspective of the person I am trying to help? How might my actions be interpreted by this person?

For further guidance and resources see the 'Care Fit for VIPS' Tool Kit at carefitforvips.co.uk (accessed 14 December 2016)

persons for what they are' – valuing their capacity *to be* rather than to do or think. This encapsulates an important view in the care context as it allows for difference, without a value judgement being placed upon that difference. From this, the fundamental duty to respect others should be independent of a person's personal characteristics and be afforded to all humans equally, regardless of their merit or ability.

Valuing People Now (DH, 2009) is one example where policy aspired to reinforce the value of respect for persons and set out to influence the ethos of services and practitioners working with people with learning disabilities and challenging behaviour. Its vision was based in the premise that:

'... all people with a learning disability are people first with the right to lead their lives like any others, with the same opportunities and responsibilities, and to be treated with the same dignity and respect. They and their families and carers are entitled to the same aspirations and life chances as other citizens.'

(DH, 2009, p.3)

This vision reflects an understanding of mutual respect for persons where all people are of equal worth and their lives, regardless of difference, are equally valuable. Despite reports of discrimination, poor access to services, abuse and neglect of individuals with learning disabilities (DH, 2012b; Mencap, 2007; Michael, 2008) and the slow progress made in delivering change following the Winterbourne View Review (Bubb, 2014), examples of good practice take account of the value of respect for persons, their humanity and dignity and provide person-centred care (DH, 2012d). The Royal College of Nursing (RCN, 2013) guidance is based on the users' experiences of healthcare and is relevant to any practitioner who cares for people with learning disabilities, regardless of the practice setting. The examples of 'positive experiences' clearly reflect a 'valuing persons' approach, whilst also suggesting ways to improve and provide dignity-enhancing care.

Respect for persons and dignity give rise to other duties, including respect for privacy. However, the relationship between respect for persons and dignity is often taken for granted. Whilst they are interrelated, it is important to understand the contribution made by the concept of dignity to value-based practice.

THE MORAL VALUE OF DIGNITY

The notion of dignity has become a dominant feature in contemporary accounts of healthcare. Appeals to the concept of dignity abound in the media and in legal, religious, political and ethical debate, with claims of 'rights to dignity', to be treated in 'a dignified way', to 'die with dignity' (Tadd, Bayer and Dieppe, 2002). Yet dignity has been criticised as an elusive and useless concept (Macklin, 2003), because it is difficult to specify what the value of dignity requires in ethical reasoning that is independent of the value of respect for persons and their autonomy (Schroeder, 2010). Häyry (2004) reminds us that although dignity is a multifaceted concept, its use can lead to constructive dialogue between people and cultures. Thus various attempts have been made to specify the concept of dignity as a value in its own right.

Given the number of inquiries and reports over recent years highlighting cases of inhumane and *undignified care*, it has become even more important to have a clear appreciation of what dignified care requires (Commission on Dignity in Care for Older People, 2012; RCN, 2013). The starting point for this is to explore how dignity may be defined and what the value of dignity entails.

Defining dignity

Nordenfelt (2004) proposed four types of dignity in his research investigating the care of older Europeans. He distinguishes types of dignity according to their position on a value scale: one that has *intrinsic worth* (that belongs to us by virtue of our nature of being *Homo sapiens*, oriented toward reason and freedom) and three with *contingent worth* (conditional on other factors; conferred on us by certain attributes, good fortune or personal merit; in some sense 'accidental' to who we are). These are further specified through their relationship with the notions of rights, respect and self-respect. The resulting four types of dignity identified by Nordenfelt (2004) are shown in *Box 5.4*.

What is common to all of these types of dignity is that the person's dignity is worthy of self-respect as well as the respect of others. They may all be evident in healthcare, although 'dignity as merit' and 'dignity as moral stature' are less relevant, as healthcare practitioners should treat people with respect for their dignity regardless of any perception of merit or moral status. These may have initially been called into question in *Case study 5.1* if Alfred was considered to be less deserving of respect or had in some way forfeited his right to be respected due to his behaviour towards another. Yet, the

BOX — **5.4**

Nordenfelt's four types of dignity

Dignity of **Menschenwürde** *(intrinsic)* – *Menschenwürde*, German for 'human worth', signifies a universal dignity that pertains to all human beings to the same extent 'just because we are all humans' and cannot be lost as long as the persons exist.

Dignity of merit (contingent) – linked to position in society; there are many kinds of this dignity and it is unevenly distributed among human beings. Dignity of merit exists by degree and can come and go. People have rights on the basis of holding certain roles or office or because they have earned merit through their actions.

Dignity of moral stature (contingent) – comes as a result of the individual's moral deeds; emerging from actions or omissions and from the kind of person he or she is. Similarly it can be reduced or lost through immoral deeds. This links with having a 'dignified character' and dignity as a virtue. The dignity of moral stature is a dignity of degree and is unevenly distributed.

Dignity of personal identity (contingent) – reflects the integrity of the person's body and mind; often, although not always, dependent on the person's self-image. It relates to one's identity as a person, to self-respect and to concepts such as autonomy and inclusion. This dignity can come and go as a result of the actions of others or as a result of changes in the person's body and mind. Thus, this kind of dignity can be violated by physical intrusion, being treated as an object or by emotional or psychological interference, for example, being humiliated or insulted.

From Nordenfelt, 2004, pp.71–9.

ACTIVITY — **5.6**

Reflecting on types of dignity in healthcare

Look at Nordenfelt's four types of dignity (*Box 5.4*).

Which do you think have most relevance to patients or service users in your care setting?

Can you identify examples where any of the types of dignity have been compromised or enhanced through your practice? Write down some examples.

inalienable, universal human dignity ('*Menschenwürde*') gives rise to due respect for our dignity simply because of our humanity, an absolute inner worth and the basic human right to be treated equally.

The *dignity of identity* is most relevant in the context of illness and disability where our personal identity and self-esteem may fluctuate due to ill-health or treatment, or may be threatened by medical intervention or care practices that invade our personal space or alter our personal identity (Killmister, 2010). Illness or disabilities may result in changes in identity over time, may restrict abilities to be autonomous or personal identity may be threatened through inadequate support or poor environment.

Jacobson (2007; 2009) views dignity as encompassing two distinct (though related) phenomena: *human dignity* and *social dignity*. *Human dignity* is the value belonging to everyone simply by virtue of being human (like Nordenfelt's universal dignity), whereas *social dignity* is generated through the interactions between individuals, groups, and societies. *Social dignity* is divided into two types: *dignity-of-self* and *dignity-in-relation*. 'Dignity-of-self' consists in the personal qualities of self-respect and self-worth, demonstrated through individual characteristics like self-confidence, integrity and *being dignified*. 'Dignity-in-relation' is concerned with the ways in which respect and worth are evident in individual and collective behaviour. Thus, expectations of dignity may depend on the moral values, beliefs and traditions of particular societies or cultures (Jacobson, 2009, p.1538).

'Dignity-in-relation' has specific relevance in healthcare because as practitioners we should uphold personal and professional values and standards of behaviour and avoid humiliation in our interactions with others as part of the obligations we afford one another as bearers of dignity (Killmister, 2010, p.160). Recognising the distinction between *dignity as a constraint* and *dignity as empowerment* is significant here (Beyleveld and Brownsword, 2001, cited by Nuffield Council on Bioethics, 2009, p.32). Certain actions may be absolutely forbidden because they are counter to human dignity (using the value of dignity as a constraint). However, thinking about dignity may also empower individuals as it supports the value of respect for persons and the obligation to treat people in ways that uphold their value as a human being.

Dignity and rights

In law and politics, the value of dignity is often interconnected with human rights. For example, the Universal Declaration of Human Rights (1948) attributes dignity to all human beings, with no reference to possession of particular conditions or qualities and starts from the assumption that it is an inalienable right that must be respected and protected. The rights arising from the Declaration apply simply because we are human beings, and would include those without capacity for rational thought.

Similarly, the importance of upholding the dignity of individuals is enshrined in UK law through the Human Rights Act (1998) which places dignity and the expectation that everyone should be treated equally, whatever their circumstances, at the heart of human rights.

These declarations of rights accord with the common use of the value of dignity in healthcare; the expectation that all people, regardless of difference or diversity, are worthy of respect and that we should practise in ways that uphold their dignity and self-worth. Dignity is not something that can be given to people in care, but neither must it be compromised or diminished through the healthcare system or care relationship (Levenson, 2007).

People's personal views of dignity

Although there are a number of formal interpretations of dignity, what matters most in the care relationship is understanding what dignity means to individuals and the value they place on maintaining and upholding their dignity in their experience of healthcare. Complete *Activity 5.7* to establish your personal viewpoint on the value of dignity.

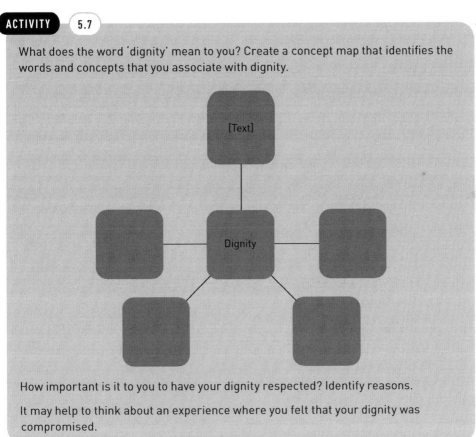

ACTIVITY 5.7

What does the word 'dignity' mean to you? Create a concept map that identifies the words and concepts that you associate with dignity.

[Text]

Dignity

How important is it to you to have your dignity respected? Identify reasons.

It may help to think about an experience where you felt that your dignity was compromised.

Although the value of dignity in itself can be hard to define, what is clear is that people recognise, and can experience significant harms, when they have not been treated with respect and due consideration for their dignity (Healthcare Commission, 2007; PHSO, 2011; Social Care Institute for Excellence (SCIE), 2006). The Health Ombudsman's Report (PHSO, 2011) provides a salutary reminder of the effect of 'casual indifference' to the values of care, respect, dignity and compassion:

> '... Older people are left in soiled or dirty clothes and are not washed or bathed. One woman told us that her aunt was taken on a long journey to a care home by ambulance. She arrived strapped to a stretcher and soaked with urine, dressed in unfamiliar clothing held up by paper clips, accompanied by bags of dirty laundry, much of which was not her own. Underlying such acts of carelessness and neglect is a casual indifference to the dignity and welfare of older patients. That this should happen anywhere must cause concern; that it should take place in a setting intended to deliver care is indefensible. The NHS must close the gap between the promise of care and compassion outlined in its Constitution and the injustice that many older people experience.'
>
> (PHSO, 2011, p.10)

The 'Dignity and Older Europeans Study' set out to establish how older people across Europe view dignity in their lives and how health and social care practitioners observe dignity when planning and providing elderly care services (Tadd, 2004; Tadd, Vanlaere and Gastmans, 2010; Woolhead *et al.*, 2004). The researchers examined the perceptions of older people from a range of different socioeconomic backgrounds, levels of health and disability, living in both institutional and community settings. Dignity was viewed as a multi-faceted concept (Woolhead *et al.*, 2004), involving:

- dignity of identity (self-respect/esteem, integrity, trust);
- human rights (equality, choice); and
- autonomy (independence, control).

Dignity was clearly important in the everyday lives of older people and, when experienced, enhanced their self-worth, self-esteem and wellbeing. However, they tended to identify dignity mostly through describing situations where they felt it was absent or jeopardised rather than enhanced.

Woolhead *et al.* (2004) found evidence of humiliation, poor communication, exclusion and a general insensitivity to their needs. Older people experienced loss of self-esteem from being treated as an 'object' and being patronised and excluded from decision-making. They were concerned about maintaining their autonomy and remaining independent, without being lonely or lacking support. They felt an inability to trust others and an increased vulnerability. Equality was important but they felt government policies did not support their rights. Woolhead *et al.* (2004) concluded that age discrimination for eligibility to services needed addressing and highlighted the need to balance care and support with promoting independence. Dignity for older people was most likely to be respected through person-centred care which focuses on communication, privacy, personal identity and feelings of vulnerability.

Tadd, Vanlaere and Gastmans (2010) use Nordenfelt's (2004) four types of dignity in their analysis of responses from the 'Older European' study and found that the *dignity of identity* raised most concern for the older people studied. Frailty, disability, illness and the ageing process may affect their identity, not only in looks but through impairments to their independence and autonomy. Ageist stereotypes can marginalise older people and make them question their value in society. With retirement and changes in their economic contribution to society, they lose not only their employment but also a sense of their identity, leading to social exclusion and isolation.

Participants wanted to be their own person with freedom and choice for as long as possible. Care supporting daily living activities and preventing burden on relatives must be balanced against fear of losing independence and choice through the interference of health and social care services. They wanted to retain control over decisions about their care and valued being informed. Poor communication, patronising and disrespectful language and manner threatened their dignity of identity while kindness, willingness to listen and politeness were valued attitudes (Tadd, Vanlaere and Gastmans, 2010).

Although these studies focused on older people, the findings start to inform what might be expected of respectful and dignified care practice for any person and in any setting.

RESPECT, DIGNITY AND PRIVACY IN PRACTICE

Defining dignity in practice

Dignity is a complex and multifactorial concept and practitioners, patients and service users may use the term in ill-defined ways. Dignity could be a subjective concept; different people may have particular understandings of when their dignity is respected or not. What is experienced as undignified care by one may be acceptable to another. Respecting dignity could become a futile objective without some consensus on a working definition and clarifying what dignity entails in practice (Tadd, 2005).

Whilst respect for persons is one of the defining attributes of the concept of dignity, it also includes privacy, autonomy and self-worth. Johnstone (2009, p.175) identifies the following elements which should inform a definition of dignity in practice:
- The intrinsic, inalienable moral worth of persons which gives rise to a duty of respect (for persons and for their humanity)
- Maintaining individuals' sense of self-worth, self-respect and self-esteem

- Respect for the autonomy of persons and as beings capable of exercising self-determination
- Supporting individuals in their exercise of autonomy, within the realms of their capabilities.

These core elements are evident in the working definitions of 'dignity' that have been presented by professional and sectoral organisations for nursing and social care (see *Box 5.5*).

BOX — 5.5

Defining dignity in care

Social Care Institute for Excellence in the SCIE Guide 15 'Dignity in Care' (first published 2006, updated 2013) uses:

'... A state, quality or manner worthy of esteem or respect; and (by extension) self-respect. Dignity in care, therefore, means the kind of care, in any setting, which supports and promotes, and does not undermine, a person's self-respect regardless of any difference. Or, as one person receiving care put it more briefly, "being treated like I was somebody".' (Policy Research Institute on Ageing and Ethnicity, 2001)

Skills for Care (2013, p.4) define dignity in the introduction to their seven common core principles to support dignity in adult social care, as:

'Dignity focuses on the significance and value of every person as a unique individual. We show our commitment to upholding other people's dignity by the ways in which we treat them; fairly, truthfully and with care and compassion. We respect others' views, choices and decisions and do not make assumptions about what they want, like or how they want to be treated... Dignity embodies the belief that everybody has equal worth and is entitled to be treated respectfully. Each individual, regardless of age, ability to consent, gender or disability, should be valued and treated as if they were able to think, feel and act in a way that would uphold their own self-respect and dignity.'

The Royal College of Nursing (RCN, 2008) defines dignity as:

'... concerned with how people feel, think and behave in relation to the worth or value of themselves and others. To treat someone with dignity is to treat them as being of worth, in a way that is respectful of them as valued individuals.'

Matiti and Baillie (2011) summarise further key themes essential to the understanding of a concept of dignity in healthcare practice:
- Dignity is inherent in human beings
- Dignity is an *internal quality*: related to self-concept, self-identity, individuality
- Dignity is *dynamic*: people adjust their perceptions of dignity as illness progresses or during hospitalisation

- Dignity has *an affective component*: it *relates to feelings* such as self-esteem, self-worth, pride, hope, confidence, self-respect, wellbeing, feeling important and valuable, comfortable
- Dignity relates to *behaviour* (and attitudes): behaving according to one's personal standards, courteousness, conveying respect, treating people as individuals and as competent adults
- Dignity is *relational*: it can be reciprocal and interpersonal
- Dignity as a sense of *personal control*: relates to autonomy, self-determination and independence
- *Presentation of self* in public: physical identity, modesty
- Dignity involves *privacy*: maintaining one's personal boundaries and space, being in control of one's privacy, respect for and protecting privacy.

(Adapted from Matiti and Baillie, 2011, pp.15–16)

Keep these different features of dignity in mind whilst completing the activity in *Case Study 5.2*, which requires you to think carefully about the values of respect for persons, dignity and privacy in your practice.

Older people may use strategies to maintain a sense of self-worth and meaning in their lives, such as focusing on simple pleasures and maintaining their sense of normality, having connections with their families and remembering their previous lives and achievements. However, dignity can be undermined by the attitudes and approaches of health and care workers in their everyday interactions with people in their care (Tadd, Vanlaere and Gastmans, 2010; Tadd *et al.*, 2011).

This was clearly evident for Barbara in *Case study 5.2*, with inappropriate and insensitive care impacting on her dignity of identity (wrong clothes, change in hairstyle) and in respect for her as a person and her universal human dignity (through the use of flippant, discourteous and condescending language, denial of personal space to meet with relatives). Reinforcing the negative aspects of the person's situation, such as their vulnerability, dependency and fragility, can make them feel insignificant and unrecognised as individuals, which, in turn, compromises their self-respect, self-esteem and dignity (Tadd, 2004; Tadd, Vanlaere and Gastmans, 2010; Woolhead *et al.*, 2004).

Jacobson (2009) suggests any human interaction between individuals or groups can be a *'dignity encounter'*, in which dignity is either violated or promoted. She identifies a number of attitudes and behaviours that can violate a patient's dignity in healthcare. These include rudeness, indifference, condescension, dismissal, disregard, dependence, intrusion, objectification, restriction, labelling, contempt, discrimination, revulsion, deprivation, assault, and abjection (being forced to compromise closely held beliefs, e.g. practices considered unclean). When a person's dignity is violated it can result in a number of potential harms to the individual (and to others in connection or relationships

CASE STUDY 5.2

Barbara and residential care

You are visiting your mother, Barbara, who is 82 years old. She is dependent on a wheelchair for mobility and has recently chosen to move into a residential home as she was finding it increasingly difficult to cope on her own (you are her only close relative and live some distance away). When you arrive she is sitting in the main living room. She is wearing clothes you do not recognise and her hair appears to have been blow-dried (for as long as you can remember she has always had a weekly 'shampoo and set'). She is normally chatty, cheerful and pleased to see you but today she is tearful and agitated.

You ask a member of staff if there is a room where you can take your mother to talk (she shares a room with two other women and one is already resting in the room). They say that all the other rooms are occupied and suggest you simply move to the other corner of the sitting room away from the television. They seem to stay nearby as if to hear what you are saying to each other.

Your mother reveals tearfully that when she was taking her daily bath that morning, one of the male care assistants had entered the bathroom to get a commode and trolley that were stored in the corner of the room. The female member of staff assisting your mother had made light of the incident, saying light-heartedly, 'Barbara, fancy your "boyfriend" coming to see you in the bath!'. Your mother is obviously upset but says the young woman meant no malice and urges you not to make a fuss.

- What issues are there to be considered here in relation to respect, dignity and privacy? As well as specific aspects of care practice, think also about other features, such as the care environment.

- What would you do differently in this situation?

- Having thought about the importance of maintaining respect and dignity in this case, make a list of ways in which you can practise to ensure that your care respects individuals and maintains their dignity.

Discuss your list with a colleague and add any new ideas that emerge from your conversation.

- Now find out whether there is a dignity policy in your work environment. If there is, read it and make notes of the key principles to be observed in your workplace.

with them) which can be physical, emotional, psychological, social, relational, spiritual and moral in nature.

Dignity is more likely to be violated if one or more of the following exists in the care relationship (Jacobson, 2009, p.1538):

- When the person (patient) is *vulnerable*, for example because of illness, helplessness, confusion or belonging to an oppressed group

- If the carer or practitioner is in *a position of antipathy*, is arrogant, hostile or impatient
- Where the care relationship is *unbalanced and unequal* – where someone, for example a practitioner, carer or relative, is in a position of greater power, authority, knowledge, or strength
- Where *practice settings* are hierarchical and rigid, where there are distractions, stress and urgency and lack of resources.

Whilst the physical environment and culture of an organisation can affect delivery of care (RCN, 2008), the values, attitudes and behaviours of individual practitioners play the most significant role in the patient's experience of dignified care (see *Box 5.6*).

BOX 5.6

RCN definition of dignity in practice (2008)

'... In care situations, dignity may be promoted or diminished by: the physical environment; organisational culture; by the attitudes and behaviour of the nursing team and others and by the way in which care activities are carried out. When dignity is present people feel in control, valued, confident, comfortable and able to make decisions for themselves. When dignity is absent people feel devalued, lacking control and comfort. They may lack confidence and be unable to make decisions for themselves. They may feel humiliated, embarrassed or ashamed. Dignity applies equally to those who have capacity and to those who lack it. Everyone has equal worth as human beings and must be treated as if they are able to feel, think and behave in relation to their own worth or value. The nursing team should, therefore, treat all people in all settings and of any health status with dignity, and dignified care should continue after death.'

The professionals involved in the 'Dignity and Older Europeans Study' viewed dignified care as that which

'... promotes autonomy, independence, engenders respect, maintains individual identity, encourages involvement, involves effective communication and is person-centred and holistic.'

(Tadd, Vanlaere and Gastmans, 2010, p.269).

Barriers to delivering dignified care included aspects of governance, protocols and staffing. Nurses recognised that patient-centred care was integral to respecting an individual's dignity, yet these behaviours were rarely seen in practice (Tadd *et al.*, 2011). Similarly, Matiti (2002) found that practitioners identified the importance of privacy for a person's dignity, yet did not see themselves as intruders of the patient's privacy. They appeared to see the care relationship as giving certain permissions to disregard respect for an individual's privacy and the usual boundaries of personal space. Yet the value of privacy is a fundamental component of dignity and can too easily be violated through inconsiderate care.

The value of privacy

Respect for persons is not only concerned with dignity and self-worth. It is also closely associated with respect for privacy. Although privacy may be an essential aspect for preserving dignity, the two concepts are quite distinct. A simple definition of privacy would be 'freedom from unauthorised intrusion' (DH, 2010b). However, privacy can be viewed in a number of ways.

Beauchamp and Childress (2013, p.312) and Allen (2011 and 2011a) identify several forms of privacy that involve limited access to the person:
* *Informational privacy* – limiting access to or keeping information about the person private
* *Physical privacy* – focuses on personal space, solitude, bodily modesty and bodily integrity; expectations that you will not be needlessly touched or exposed
* *Locational privacy* – focuses on environment, having control and choice of one's surroundings
* *Decisional privacy* – concerned with autonomy and personal choices in healthcare decision-making; for example, reproductive decisions including contraception, abortion, assisted reproductive technology; choosing medically unhealthy lifestyles; the right to refuse care
* *Proprietary privacy* – 'property interests' of the person; privacy of the body; self-ownership and control over personal identifiers such as keeping their image private, genetic data and body tissues
* *Relational or associational privacy* – concerned with the relationships within which people make decisions with significant others, such as families or intimate relationships. This would include intimate sharing of their experience of death, illness and recovery.

Individuals generally value their bodily modesty, intimacy and bodily integrity. Most patients tend to be discreet and reserved when sharing sensitive health information (Allen, 2011a) and would expect the same from practitioners.

Normally restrictions are placed on access to health information and the law imposes obligations to respect informational privacy through the Data Protection Act (1998). However, preserving privacy is too narrowly construed if the focus is on one or other of these forms of privacy, and all forms identified above should be taken into account when devising policy and care strategies. Conditions of access to the person should be agreed in relation to what will constitute the violation of their right to privacy. Practitioners should respect the person's privacy (in all its forms); their bodily modesty, intimacy, bodily integrity, and self-ownership (Allen, 2011a).

Privacy in practice

You may think about privacy from a very practical viewpoint; for example, maintaining privacy by drawing curtains when meeting patients' hygiene needs or knocking on doors before entering cubicles. You could also identify with the underlying moral values related to maintaining privacy, such as establishing a relationship of trust, the importance of respecting the person, treating them as an individual and promoting and supporting their independence. All of these perspectives are important in developing and enhancing your practice, as you need to think not only about what you should do but also the value associated with practising in a certain way.

You will have recognised violation of a number of aspects of a person's privacy in *Case study 5.2* and identified different approaches that would demonstrate respect for Barbara as a person and provide care in a way that maintains her individuality and protects her privacy. It is often in the fundamental aspects of care, such as meeting hygiene needs, that dignity, respect and privacy can be most at risk. This is particularly relevant if care becomes routinised and you underestimate the importance of the aspects of care that are taken for granted. Practitioners must be wary of becoming desensitised to some of the expectations placed on people in their care.

The reality for people requiring care in hospitals, care homes or in their own homes is that they will inevitably expose themselves, both physically and emotionally, to practitioners and carers in ways that would not occur in their normal everyday lives. Sleeping in rooms with other people, sharing bathing and toilet facilities, using commodes with only the 'protection' of a flimsy curtain, discussing personal thoughts, feelings and intimate information with relative strangers in the process of assessment and diagnosis are all examples that can compromise a person's privacy and challenge their ability to maintain their self-respect and dignity.

There will inevitably be times when total privacy cannot be maintained. However, you should seek permission from the patient wherever possible and must be able to justify any compromise of privacy, both on practical grounds and in terms of the person's moral right to privacy. It is essential that you take responsibility for safeguarding the privacy and dignity of patients and service users in your delivery of care.

In their research with cardiothoracic patients, Whitehead and Wheeler (2008) set out to ascertain the patients' experience of how they thought their privacy needs were met, and how the care environment could enhance the patients' privacy during their hospital stay. The key themes that patients identified reflect the different types of privacy identified by Beauchamp and Childress (2013) and Allan (2011). They also start to identify what kinds of approaches would be important to protecting the privacy of people in your care (see *Box 5.7*).

BOX 5.7

Patients' concept and definition of privacy

Important themes for patients included:

- Privacy of information, e.g. one's conversation not being overheard
- Privacy of person and body, e.g. not being viewed during one's private moments
- Exerting personal control, e.g. matters relating to one's care
- Able to be alone at one's choosing
- Gain respect from professionals
- Having one's hospital records and files removed from visitors' attention/space
- Having one's own personal space
- Everyone valuing privacy as essential
- The value of single as opposed to mixed-sex wards/bays
- Freedom and privacy to worship
- Right to perform intimate activities of daily living, e.g. using the toilet, in private and alone, only having staff present if essential.

Adapted from Whitehead, J. and Wheeler, H. (2008) Patients' experience of privacy and dignity. Part 2: an empirical study, *British Journal of Nursing*, **17(7)**: 458–464.

One of the common patient experiences where a person's dignity and privacy are at risk of compromise, is in the performance of intimate personal care, such as washing and assistance with using the toilet or continence care (see *Activity 5.8*).

ACTIVITY 5.8

Privacy and dignity in continence care

- Reflect on how you would feel if you were dependent on others for aspects of your own personal care, such as washing, going to the toilet and managing your continence.

For applications of values of respect, dignity and privacy in practice see the reports from the 'Privacy and Dignity in Continence Care Project' (Centre for Health Services Studies, British Geriatrics Society and Royal College of Physicians, 2009) at rcplondon.ac.uk/projects/continence-care-privacy-dignity or kar.kent. ac.uk/24800/1/Phase_1_Privacy_and_Dignity_in_Continence_Care_Report_ November_2009.pdf

- Think about your current practice in relation to continence care:
  - Are there things that you could do better?
  - How will you achieve these goals?
  - How will you know when you have been successful in improving your care?

Pols (2013) examined different interpretations of dignity in care practices in psychiatric hospitals and residential homes and carers' views about 'good care', including the washing of patients. She found that, '... geriatric assistants enforced cleanliness far too routinely for the taste of the psychiatric nurses who came to work in the residential homes' (p. 191). The latter preferred approaches that allowed residents to influence the organisation of their washing practices, whereas for the geriatric assistants, '... washing patients was never questioned: it simply needed to be done' (Pols, 2013).

ACTIVITY ⟨ **5.9** ⟩

Read pages 191–7 of Pols' (2013) article and make notes from her analysis of why there were differences in expectations of practice between the two different groups of practitioners and settings and their ways of achieving dignity.

Pols, J. (2013) Washing the patient: dignity and aesthetic values in nursing care. *Nursing Philosophy*, **14(3):** 186–200.

What is evident from Pols' (2013) study is that practitioners working in multidisciplinary teams may have different philosophical standpoints of what constitutes care, dignity and respect and how this should be achieved. This in part can relate to them as individuals, to the organisational or practice setting and to differences in role and professional discipline.

Protecting and promoting respect, dignity and privacy in practice

Ensuring that respect, privacy and dignity are protected and promoted is everyone's responsibility. It is therefore essential that you observe professional standards and policies put in place to ensure this. However, this is only the first step to understanding the value of respect for others and to preventing circumstances in which a patient's privacy and dignity may be infringed. You need the knowledge, skills and values that will enable you to practise with sensitivity. Also, if you are serious about the importance of respect for persons and dignity in your care then it is essential that you are not lulled into a false sense of security provided by simply claiming to follow routines, protocols and guidelines. Observing these is only the first step to being committed to seeing, understanding and knowing the value of respect for others and to prevent behaviour and attitudes that degrade, devalue and humiliate individuals in your care.

As Levenson (2007, p.14) states:

'... Dignity is not a formula or a recipe that can be rigidly applied from a manual. In particular, the 'toolkit' approach, while useful for improving practice and as a benchmark for assessing performance, cannot fully address the 'care' component of dignity in care. Indeed, a formulaic approach, taken outside the context of values and principles, can lead to a situation where all the right boxes are ticked, but still standards fall short of what older people (and other age groups too) want.' (p.14).

She identified a number of core principles that underlie dignity in care (*Box 5.8*).

BOX 5.8

Core principles that underlie dignity in care

- Dignity in care is inseparable from the wider context of dignity as a whole
- Dignity is about treating people as individuals
- Dignity is not just about physical care
- Dignity thrives in the context of equal power relationships
- Dignity must be actively promoted (rather than simply attempting to eradicate indignity)
- Dignity is more than the sum of its parts.

From Levenson, 2007, p.13.

In a survey conducted for the Royal College of Nursing (Baillie, Gallagher and Wainwright, 2008), respondents identified care activities that can compromise an individual's dignity, including many physical aspects of care such as personal care, procedures involving intimate areas of the body or that were potentially painful or anxiety-provoking, as well as aspects of mental healthcare and care involving emotions. The main factors identified in either promoting or diminishing dignity in care were grouped according to *the 'three Ps'*:
- *'Place'* (physical environment and organisational culture)
- *'Process'* (the nature and conduct of care activities)
- *'People'* (attitudes and behaviours of staff and others).

Reflecting on the factors that impact on the 'three Ps' should help you to identify the specific aspects of practice essential in providing respectful and dignified care in your care setting and any changes that need to be made to improve the patient and service user experience. The RCN Dignity 'pocket guide' provides a useful summary of practical ideas in providing dignified care grouped according to the 'three Ps' (available at rcn.org.uk/professional-development/publications/pub-003292 (accessed 14 December 2016).

Respect for persons and their dignity is most likely to be achieved through inclusive and person-centred approaches to care which focus on personal identity, promoting

ACTIVITY 5.10

Preserving and promoting dignity and privacy in healthcare

1. Reflect on your own practice and identify which people are most vulnerable to loss of dignity and why this is the case.

2. How might you work to protect or minimise loss of dignity when you are caring for these people? What are the key aspects and approaches in your practice

   that are important in providing dignified care? You should have some ideas that you can take from your list created in response to *Case study 5.2*.

3. Think about and list the key aspects and approaches you identify according to the categories of 'Place', 'Process' and 'People'.

4. Discuss your list with a group of practitioners and refine your 'guide' to preserving and promoting dignity and privacy in your care setting.

5. Identify **one aspect of practice** where you could make a simple change today that would maximise positive impact on patient or service user dignity.

Useful sources include:

Baillie, Gallagher and Wainwright (2008) *'Defending Dignity: challenges and opportunities for nursing'* on the RCN website at rcn.org.uk/professional-development/publications/pub-003257 (accessed 14 December 2016)

Commission on Dignity in Care for Older People (collaboration established by the NHS Confederation, the Local Government Association and Age UK) (2012) *Delivering Dignity. Securing dignity in care for older people in hospitals and care homes. Final Report.*

Jackson, A. and Irwin, W. (2011) Dignity, humanity and equality: Principle of Nursing Practice A. *Nursing Standard*, **25(28):** 35–37.

Essence of Care 2010 – benchmarks for the fundamental aspects of care (DH, 2010b) particularly the section 'Privacy and Dignity' and the indicators for best practice identified by patients, carers and professionals.

autonomy and enhancing privacy, using respectful communication and building caring relationships that recognise human rights such as fairness and equality (Tadd *et al.*, 2011). The individual must be seen as central and any feelings of vulnerability recognised and addressed (see *Box 5.9*).

The Dignity in Care campaign, launched in November 2006, aims to place dignity and respect at the heart of UK care services (National Dignity Council, 2015). The campaign has over 70 000 registered 'Dignity Champions' (as at April 2016), who work individually and collectively to ensure people have a good care experience.

Patients' views of how their dignity needs might be met

- Absence of embarrassment, e.g. not shown up in front of others
- Having one's privacy and dignity respected
- Being treated humanely, like a human being and not as an object
- Being treated with respect as well as respecting others
- Being treated with sympathy, consideration and compassion
- To be treated as an individual
- Staff introducing themselves and saying who they are before treating you
- Being able to maintain one's privacy, e.g. treated in private, out of public gaze
- A feeling of being in control, e.g. over decisions and private bodily functions
- Staff explaining treatment, any changes and what is going to happen
- Being listened to and being heard
- Desire to have own personal space and independence
- Acknowledgement of the need for peace of mind at a stressful time.

Adapted from Whitehead and Wheeler, 2008, p.461.

ACTIVITY — 5.11

Being a Dignity Champion

If the term 'champion' is used to describe someone who is a 'defender', a 'supporter' and a 'campaigner' (as well as a 'remarkable person', someone demonstrating 'excellence') what *qualities* would you expect a 'Dignity Champion' to have?

Find out how to become a Dignity Champion and the qualities required at dignityincare.org.uk/Dignity-Champions/Becoming_a_Dignity_Champion/ (accessed 16 December 2016)

The '*10 Dignity Do's*' (previously the 10 Point Dignity Challenge) (Dignity in Care, 2015) describe the values and actions that should be expected of high quality services in respecting people's dignity. They should:

1. Have a zero tolerance of all forms of abuse
2. Support people with the same respect you would want for yourself or a member of your family
3. Treat each person as an individual by offering a personalised service
4. Enable people to maintain the maximum possible level of independence, choice and control
5. Listen and support people to express their needs and wants

6. Respect people's right to privacy
7. Ensure people feel able to complain without fear of retribution
8. Engage with family members and carers as care partners
9. Assist people to maintain confidence and positive self-esteem
10. Act to alleviate people's loneliness and isolation.

Good interpersonal and communication skills, both verbal and non-verbal, are essential to respectful and personalised care. They include interactions that promote dignity through helping people to feel comfortable in the care relationship, in control and valued as individuals (see *Table 5.1*).

Table 5.1 *Interactions that make patients feel comfortable, in control and valued*

Interactions that help people feel comfortable	• Sensitivity • Empathy • Developing relationships • Conversation • Professionalism • Family involvement (if desired by the patient) • Friendliness and reassurance • Humour (if used sensitively and appropriately)
Communication that helps people feel in control	• Giving explanations and information • Providing informed consent • Offering choices and negotiating • Enabling independence
Communication that helps people to feel valued	• Listening • Giving time • Showing concern for patients as individuals • Being kind, considerate and helpful • Showing courtesy: addressing people by their preferred name, introducing self, being polite and respectful, including respect for culture and religious beliefs

Source: Baillie and Black, 2015, p.125, originally adapted by Baillie and Black from Baillie, 2007 and RCN, 2008.

The Health Foundation (2014) identifies examples of practical tools to support dignity in care. These include:

- introducing yourself by name and profession (the *'Hello my name is'* campaign)
- using *one-page patient profiles* as a focused strategy to getting to know what is important to the patient and the personalisation of their care
- gathering *patient stories and shadowing patients* on their care pathway, observing and recording what happens, and seeking their feedback on each step

BOX — **5.10**

Practice notes – enablers of respectful and dignified care

- Be self-aware and develop courteous, respectful communication and interpersonal skills, including active listening, politeness, allowing time for provision of information, for understanding, and questions.
- Act fairly, compassionately and sensitively.
- Introduce yourself and ask individuals how they would prefer to be addressed, i.e. first name, surname, family name, etc.
- Ask for consent to share information with other carers.
- Where possible, orientate individuals to their environment including information about quiet areas, privacy and confidentiality.
- Ensure the physical environment takes account of specific needs including appropriate signage, careful use of colour, information and date boards, safe walking spaces and communal areas to improve social interaction and engagement.
- Provide gender-specific facilities; for example, wards, toilets and washing facilities.
- Take account of personal preferences, lifestyle choices and cultural factors when assessing their needs and providing support for care.
- Ensure people receive care or treatment in a dignified way that does not embarrass, humiliate or expose them; this includes the way information is exchanged at the bedside or in other communal environments.
- Don't make assumptions about appropriate standards of hygiene or appearance for individuals and provide support to maintain appearance to their level of expectation, e.g. hair, standards of dress, etc. (for example, just because you shower every morning does not mean they should).
- Maintain confidentiality of personal and treatment information.
- Particular care is needed to maintain privacy when using interpreters; individuals may prefer to use a family member or the same interpreter on each occasion.
- Demonstrate respect for personal belongings, for example, access to individuals' own clothing, access to bed lockers.
- Respect privacy of personal space, for example, knocking on doors before entering rooms. Use ways to prevent being disturbed when providing care at the bedside, such as pegs and signs for curtains.
- Provide areas for private conversations, needs assessment, phone calls, etc.
- Enable individuals to personalise and make choices about their living environment, particularly in care homes.
- Be confident to challenge the negative attitudes of others and report through the appropriate channels practice that diminishes dignity.
- Be reflective – exercise critical value-based reflection on your own and others' practice.

Compiled and adapted from SCIE, 2013; DH, 2010b; Jackson and Irwin, 2011 and Tadd *et al.*, 2011a.

- implementing *Schwartz Rounds* – an approach to help providers of health and social care develop their organisational culture and support staff by allowing time for staff reflection and sharing insights.

See more at: health.org.uk/newsletter/seven-practical-tools-support-dignity-and-compassion-care (accessed 16 December 2016)

The practice notes (see *Box 5.10*) provide a summary of ways to enable the protection and promotion of respect, dignity and privacy in your practice.

CONCLUSION

Being worthy of respect and the value placed on dignity are based in our shared humanity and the intrinsic value attributed to every human being. One important implication of respect for persons and human dignity is that every person should be acknowledged as an inherently valuable member of the community and as a unique individual entitled to the same level of respect as any other. Respect for persons and human dignity should have no boundaries and go beyond any social order, such that they cannot be legitimately violated by society. In this way, respect for persons and dignity are the basis for human rights and are fundamental to our feelings of self-esteem and self-worth. What is clear is that practitioners should never take for granted the values of respect for persons and dignity nor the implications of their consideration in practice.

In this chapter you have explored the value of respect for persons as a core value and, if this is properly understood and integrated into care, many of the other values flow from it. Having respect for persons and their humanity facilitates a philosophy of care that promotes dignity for patients and service users, even in situations of great dependence. The importance placed on privacy in maintaining an individual's dignity and the need to develop care strategies that protect and promote privacy have been emphasised.

We have identified that respect for persons is associated with a number of other values such as valuing humanity, dignity and privacy. However, we have consciously separated out respect for persons and autonomy, as it is important that you recognise and remember that although they are interrelated they are also distinct. Respect for persons is a value that implies a broader set of obligations than simply respecting an individual's autonomy, which has self-determination as its main focus. The value associated with respect for autonomy is important in today's health and care practice and gives rise to a number of guiding principles and procedural aspects of care which we explore in *Chapter 6*.

CHAPTER SUMMARY

Four key points to take away from Chapter 5:

- The values of respect, dignity and privacy are fundamental to care practice.
- If respect is properly understood and integrated into care, many of the other values will flow from it.
- Having respect for persons and their humanity promotes the dignity of patients and service users, even in situations of great dependence.
- Dignity and privacy can easily be compromised if care becomes routinised; therefore you must be critically reflective of your own and others' practice and adopt enabling approaches that protect and promote the dignity and privacy of individuals in your care.

FURTHER READING

Brooker, D. and Latham, I. (2015) *Person-Centred Dementia Care: making services better with the VIPS framework*, 2nd ed. London: Jessica Kingsley.

Hughes, J.C. (2014) *How We Think About Dementia: personhood, rights, ethics, the arts and what they mean for care.* London: Jessica Kingsley.

Matiti, M.R. and Baillie, L. (2011) *Dignity in Healthcare: a practical approach for nurses and midwives.* London: Radcliffe.

06

AUTONOMY AND THE PRINCIPLE OF RESPECT FOR AUTONOMY

LEARNING OUTCOMES:

In this chapter you will:

- Identify the distinction between being autonomous and the principle of respect for autonomy

- Define personal autonomy and identify and explore the necessary conditions to be autonomous, including the notions of capacity and competence

- Examine duties and rules arising from respect for autonomy and their implications for practice

- Consider the notion of paternalism and reflect on care strategies that promote autonomy

- Explore the moral value and practice of informed consent as an expression of autonomy.

INTRODUCTION

Autonomy and the principle of respect for autonomy are fundamental values in daily life and in health and care practice. We value our personal autonomy and may also view autonomy as a right. Personal autonomy is often associated with individual choice. We generally expect to be able to choose for ourselves how we should live and act, subject to restrictions arising from the rights of others to exercise their autonomy. Intuitively, choice and personal autonomy are morally important and the principle of respect for autonomy has become accepted as an ideal in health and social care and bioethics.

In healthcare, the NHS Constitution (DH, 2015a) reflects the fundamental standards below which care must never fall and reinforces the individual's rights to respect, choice and individualised care. Patient choice is supported by the NHS Choice Framework

(DH, 2014d) and autonomy and respect are fundamental principles in the *Essence of Care* (DH, 2010b) and the RCN *Principles of Care* for nursing practice (RCN, 2011). *Valuing People Now* (DH, 2009) supports independence, choice and personalisation of care for people with learning disabilities, whilst the *Mental Health Act 1983: code of practice* (DH, 2015) emphasises the importance of empowerment, patient and carer involvement and protection of individuals' rights and autonomy. The principle of respect for autonomy supports other moral duties in practice, such as confidentiality and informed consent, which also have legal authority (GMC, 2008). Similarly, The Care Act (2014) provides the legal framework for social care which prioritises individual needs, promotes individual wellbeing and puts the person at the centre of their care with rights to choice.

The values of autonomy and respect underpin the notions of patient participation and public involvement in health (Foot *et al.*, 2014), inclusive service user involvement and advocacy (Beresford, 2013), woman-centred care in midwifery (Kirkham, 2010) and person-centred dementia care (Kitwood, 1997; Brooker, 2007; Brooker and Latham, 2015).

Before we go any further, there is an important distinction to be made here. 'Being autonomous' is a condition usually associated with individuals; our personal autonomy. Respect for autonomy is a guiding moral principle; a rule or obligation to act or practise with due respect for another person's autonomy. To understand this principle you need first to explore what it means to be autonomous.

DEFINING AUTONOMY

ACTIVITY 6.1

Your personal definition of autonomy

1. Think about and write down all the words, phrases and ideas that come to mind when you think about 'autonomy'. What does 'being autonomous' mean to you? If it helps, create a concept map:

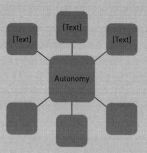

2. Look up 'autonomy' in a dictionary and add the definition to your concept map.
3. Now talk to some relatives, friends and/or colleagues about what autonomy means to them.
4. Try writing your own definition of autonomy.

You may find that you identified words and phrases similar to those already discussed in *Chapter 5*, such as a person's capacity to make choices and decisions. This is not surprising, as being autonomous and respect for autonomy are closely associated with respect for persons. If we value and respect people as individuals, then we should also respect their ability to make choices and to be in control of their own lives without undue interference from others. Autonomy is important in cultures where all individuals are considered to be unique and valued members of society.

The word 'autonomy' is derived from the Greek word *autos* meaning 'self' and *nomos* meaning 'rule, governance or law'. Different writers give alternative accounts of autonomy, although most acknowledge that autonomy incorporates the capacity for self-determination. Definitions of autonomy often include reference to:
* self-governance
* independence
* individuality
* individual choice
* freedom/freedom of will
* being one's own person.

Gerald Dworkin (1988, p.5) in his classic text *The Theory and Practice of Autonomy* reminds us that there are many interpretations of the term 'autonomy'. It may be used to mean self-rule or liberty. It is often equated with dignity, integrity, individuality, responsibility and independence, and is associated with the personal qualities of self-assertion, critical reflection and with having knowledge of one's own interests. He goes on to state that,

> '... the only features held constant ... are that autonomy is a feature of persons and that it is a desirable quality to have.'
>
> (Dworkin, 1988, p.6).

What Dworkin alludes to here is that people value their autonomy; most people see 'being autonomous' or having 'respect for an individual's autonomy' as being desirable qualities or aims. Some reasons why we value our autonomy include:
* people are usually the best judge of what is good for them, so respecting their autonomous decisions will, on the whole, contribute to their happiness and wellbeing
* being autonomous is part of human flourishing; people have a deep need to discover, create and express their own individual characters
* the value attributed to persons and the unconditional worth of humanity.

Christman (2015, s.1.1) uses the term 'basic autonomy' to mean '... the minimal status of being responsible, independent and able to speak for oneself ... and free of manipulative, self-distorting influences...'. This definition reflects the fact that most adults will be autonomous, except perhaps those who are suffering extremes of debilitating illness or from oppressive social constructs, contexts or practices. In health and care you should always start from the assumption that a person is capable of being autonomous, unless there are strong justifiable reasons to think otherwise. Autonomy is not an all or nothing concept; it is *a matter of degree*. It is possible to be autonomous in some regards or at some times and not others. We assume you would consider yourself to be autonomous, yet you may well have experienced times when you felt your usual level of autonomy was compromised; for example, in new and unfamiliar circumstances or during illness.

In addition, being autonomous is usually associated with being an adult. However, there is a significant amount of research into children's developing ability to be autonomous and their rights to be involved in decisions that impact on them as individuals and their present and future lives. If you want to read more about this, a good place to start is with work by Priscilla Alderson who writes passionately about making care decisions with children and their families (see Alderson, 2000 and 2002).

The value of autonomy

Most people would see being autonomous and having respect for autonomy as desirable qualities or aims. Autonomy can be viewed as having intrinsic value and as being instrumentally valuable, and respect for autonomy is a principle endorsed by both utilitarian and deontological positions.

Utilitarians would accept the principle of respect for autonomy, as long as exercising your autonomy or respecting autonomy does not cause harm to others. Is it in the interests of society as a whole? Does it achieve the greatest good for the greatest number? A simple utilitarian argument would be that autonomy has instrumental value because it helps to promote our happiness. People are usually the best judge of what is good for them, so respecting their autonomous decisions will, on the whole, lead to happiness. One counter-argument to this might be that this gives us little justification to respect someone's autonomous decision if it is clearly against their interests e.g. if it puts their life at serious risk.

A more sophisticated argument might suggest that the exercise of our autonomy does not so much lead to happiness but actually constitutes part of human happiness because human beings have a deep need to discover, create and express their own individual characters.

Kantian deontologists recognise the rational capacity of human beings; that individuals are ends in themselves and should not be subject to another's will. Kant argued that respect for autonomy comes from the recognition that all persons have unconditional worth, each having the capacity to determine their own destiny. For Kant, what distinguishes us from non-autonomous creatures is our ability to deliberate about our own actions and choose those that are morally right. This ability must be based in reason and not desire. This account equates the exercise of autonomy with rationality and that we ought to treat our own and others' rationality and autonomy with respect.

FORMAL DEFINITIONS AND KEY COMPONENTS OF AUTONOMY

BOX 6.1

Some formal definitions of autonomy

'Individual autonomy is an idea that is generally understood to refer to the capacity to be one's own person, to live one's life according to reasons and motives that are taken as one's own and not the product of manipulative or distorting external forces.'

(Christman, 2015, p.1)

Beauchamp and Childress (2013, pp.101–2) define personal autonomy as

'... self-rule that is free from both controlling interference by others and limitations that prevent meaningful choice, such as inadequate understanding. The autonomous individual acts freely in accordance with a self-chosen plan ... a person of diminished autonomy is in some material respect controlled by others or incapable of deliberating or acting on the basis of his or her desires and plans.'

Gillon's (1986, p.60) definition has similar requirements, in that he states that autonomy is

'...the capacity to think, decide and act on the basis of such thought and decision freely and independently and without... let or hindrance.'

There are at least four elements relevant to autonomy that are implied by the definitions in *Box 6.1*:

- the value of personhood and respect for persons
- the ability to be self-governing and to determine one's own personal goals, preferences and desires
- human agency; the capacity or competence to make choices based on our reasoning and the capacity for intentional action
- being free from controlling interferences and the freedom to act upon the choices that are made.

ACTIVITY 6.2

Imagine you are on a weight-reducing diet and you have been really pleased with your weight loss so far. However, today is turning out to be a particularly stressful day at work, so when you go for coffee you cannot resist buying a Danish pastry and a chocolate bar. You feel you deserve them, given the morning you have had but, once you have eaten them, you feel guilty and angry with yourself and wish you hadn't let yourself down in this way.

- Was choosing to eat the Danish pastry and chocolate an autonomous decision?
- How might you explain your decision and actions to another person?

In this situation deciding to eat one cake or bar of chocolate will not be disastrous for your diet. However, the question of whether you were autonomous in this decision-making helps to illustrate some of the complexities in understanding autonomy. You would probably consider yourself to be an autonomous adult and, in making a choice here, even if it was for cake and chocolate, you may feel that you were acting autonomously as this was your own individual decision. Some concept of basic autonomy might well concur with this view. However, on reflection, this might not have been your truly autonomous decision, given that you regret your choice. You may be reasoning that you succumbed to some compulsion or influence, such as the satisfaction of basic desires for pleasure and comfort, which do not accord with your ultimate, higher order aims to lose weight or eat a healthy diet.

Gillon (1986, p.61) helps us to understand a number of components of autonomy that are relevant here when he describes three types of autonomy:

* autonomy of thought
* autonomy of will
* autonomy of action.

Thinking about each of these should help you to recognise that a person's autonomy may be compromised in one or all of these areas.

Autonomy of thought

Autonomy of thought includes the wide range of intellectual skills that encompass the ability to think for oneself when deliberating about choices, preferences and wants, believing things and making decisions, such as your conscious and reasoned decision to lose weight.

Autonomy of will

Autonomy of will is the freedom to decide to do things based on your deliberations and intentions, i.e. your 'willpower'. For example, you can decide not to eat a chocolate bar despite the powerful desire to do so. However, autonomy of will may be diminished by a number of influences, either internal – for example, disease or addiction to drugs – or external, such as threats or manipulation.

Autonomy of action

Autonomy of action is acting for oneself; being able to act on the basis of one's autonomous thought and will. For example, a person with paralysis may have autonomy of thought but be restricted in their autonomy of action because they are unable to act without the assistance of others.

Each of these three forms of autonomy requires some basis in reasoning – the ability to deliberate about choices and to establish a reason for the decision or action. However, the quality or types of reasons may differ between individuals, which is important to remember when considering the choices made by patients and service users and in issues of competence.

Dworkin's (1988) account of autonomy highlights the need for individuals to have the capacity to reflect critically upon their values, preferences and desires and to endorse or change these in the light of higher order desires, such that your decisions and choices are authentically your own. This condition of personal autonomy is sometimes referred to as authenticity and a person is said to act autonomously when they act on the desires they have decided to endorse (based in reflection), and when their decision is not the result of manipulation, coercion or other controlling influences.

Dworkin presents what is known as a procedural understanding of autonomy. This is primarily concerned with the process of decision-making rather than the actual choice or decision that is reached. This is important when we talk about the process of informed consent. Procedural accounts of autonomy are often based in self-reflection, evaluative capacities and procedural independence, with limited judgement of the value of the actual content of the desires or preferences. On this account, we may feel that another person's choices are reckless or irrational from our viewpoint, but they would still be autonomous if their choices and decisions have been reached through reflection and endorsement without undue influence and are therefore their own.

So, to go back to the cake and chocolate example, it appears that you made a conscious and deliberate choice to lose weight and that this was your principal aim. It is not that this desire is better in itself; it is the fact that you have reasoned and chosen this as your primary desire or preference. However, on this occasion, you may have given way to some compulsions or 'controlling' influences, such as tiredness, stress and a basic desire for comfort. It is unlikely in this case that you were coerced, but you may have been subject to some external manipulating influences such as the positioning of chocolate and cakes close to the till point where you wait for your coffee or seeing 'special offers' if you buy the two items together. This does not mean that you lack autonomy altogether; just that your autonomy has been compromised temporarily in this particular situation.

These accounts of autonomy, which include reference to making choices on the basis of reflection on and ordering of our desires and preferences and being free from or having the ability to resist distorting or controlling influences, are particularly relevant in the context of health promotion aimed at helping individuals to change their health behaviours.

ACTIVITY 6.3

Reflection

Think of one aspect of practice where you might be expected to support an individual to change their health behaviour. This could include supporting someone with smoking cessation, advising a parent in the provision of a healthier diet for their child, working with someone who drinks excessive amounts of alcohol, encouraging safer sex practices, introducing exercise regimes following a myocardial infarction (heart attack).

- Would you consider the person/people you were working with to be fully autonomous? Explain your answer. Think about the accounts of autonomy presented by Gillon (1986) and Dworkin (1988).
- What challenges have you faced in advising or supporting the individual?
- Was their autonomy compromised in any ways?
- What kinds of influences could interfere with their autonomy?
- In completing this activity you should have started to identify that there are factors that affect whether or not an individual can be autonomous in their choices and actions.

NECESSARY CONDITIONS TO BE AUTONOMOUS

For an individual to be autonomous, requires possession of certain attributes and competencies of self-determination as well as other factors.

ACTIVITY 6.4

Reflection

Think about an important decision that you have had to make in your personal life. It could be buying or renting a new property, changing your job, or something else of significance to you.

- What decision did you have to make? What options did you have?
- What did you do to help you make a choice?
- How long did it take from first identifying the need to reach a decision to, for example, completing the purchase?
- Who else was involved in the decision-making? This may have included friends, relatives and strangers. In what ways did they influence your decision?
- Did anything hinder your final decision-making?
- Were you confident in the decision that you made? If not, explain why not.

You should see from your reflections that being autonomous can be a complex activity, particularly where we are called upon to make important, unfamiliar or demanding choices. Similar challenges confront patients and service users when they are faced with choices outside their normal realm of decision-making or where the consequences of their decisions are potentially life-changing. You should also have identified a number of factors or conditions that are necessary in order for an individual to be autonomous, both internal to the person concerned and external factors that relate to the context in which the person is functioning, and certain enabling conditions. Your list should include:

Understanding and capacity
- ability to understand and reflect on the issues involved and to 'weigh them up'; the capacity for rational thought, to make choices and decisions
- knowing yourself, your personal values, preferences, desires
- authenticity or endorsement of your desires, preferences, values that motivate your choices
- attitudes to self, such as self-respect, self-trust, self-esteem.

Voluntariness and freedom from interference
- the freedom to exercise decision-making capacities
- being able to act voluntarily, free from manipulation or coercion when making choices and decisions.

Having choices
- the nature and extent of the options available; if individuals are being asked to make choices then there must be real and meaningful options to choose from.

Information
- having adequate information on which to base the decision (this need not be all available information but should be sufficient to weigh up the harms and benefits of a particular choice and its potential consequences).

Deliberation
- having the opportunity to deliberate – allowing time to reflect on choices and to check out understanding, particularly in new contexts or unfamiliar decisions.

Environment
- being in an environment that supports and fosters autonomy; the individual must believe that their autonomous choice will be facilitated, supported and accepted.

The opportunity to exercise choice

- having made a choice, the individual must be able to put that choice into action without fear of punishment or recrimination.

BOX 6.2

Summary of necessary components of 'being autonomous'

- Rationality (minimal competency) and agency (the capacity for intentional action)
- The capacity for rational thought, knowing oneself and self-control and the competence to make choices
- Freedom to exercise these capacities: independence from controlling influences or interferences that would prevent individuals making choices for themselves
- Authenticity conditions, i.e. capacity to reflect on and endorse (or identify with) one's desires and values (e.g. Dworkin, 1988).

Influencing decisions

This section considers influences that are external to the person, such as their environment and the effect of others, including family, friends and carers. These external influences can impact on an individual's abilities for autonomous decision-making (although not always negatively).

Your role in the relationship with a patient or service user is obviously an important external influence on their autonomy. Beauchamp and Childress (2013, pp.138–9) identify three forms of influence that may exert control over another person's ability to make autonomous decisions – coercion, persuasion and manipulation. Each of these may differ in moral significance (see *Box 6.3*).

You may feel that the likelihood of coercion is minimal in healthcare. Any form of threat will erode an individual's autonomy and could cause significant harms emotionally, psychologically and physically, including the breakdown of trust in the healthcare relationship and avoidance of intervention. However, quite subtle forms of influence may be perceived as threatening by some patients and service users. For instance, if you give a patient a range of options but imply that, if they do not choose a particular one, they may lose your support, care or concern, this may easily be perceived as a threat. The environment may also be threatening and not conducive to making decisions; for example, an unfamiliar clinical environment with limited privacy. A person's choice may also be manipulated without using threat but still in ways that undermine their autonomy – a disapproving look, telling lies or evading the truth, or withholding information such as unpleasant side-effects. You will look at the value of truth-telling in *Chapter 7*.

BOX 6.3

Forms of influence

Coercion = intentional use of a credible and severe threat of harm or force to control another (where the threat is real or sufficient deceit is used to make a person believe it could be) e.g. the threat of force used by police, courts or hospitals for involuntary treatment and detention for mental health problems.

Persuasion = '... a person must come to believe in something through the merit of reasons another person advances.' i.e. influenced by appeal to reason (not emotion)

Manipulation = neither coercion or persuasion; '... swaying people to do what the manipulator wants by means other than coercion or persuasion', e.g. a deliberate act to manage the information given to a person with the intent of altering their understanding and motivate them to do what the 'manipulator' intended.

Source: Beauchamp and Childress, 2013, pp.138–9.

Hollomotz (2014) considers whether *Valuing People Now* (DH, 2009) positively influenced the decisions available to adults with learning difficulties or was just 'choice-based policy rhetoric' and tokenistic in practice. Although individuals appeared to make a range of decisions, the availability of 'mundane choices' was significantly influenced by staff. For example, people were free to choose from a menu of activities at a day centre but these activities were restricted and pre-agreed by the staff, who then retained control. Service users had limited choice as to whether they attended the day centre or did something else, such as paid employment. Thus, the individual's freedom to make decisions was manipulated and restricted by their carers, albeit on the premise of minimising risk and the desire to protect individuals from 'unwise' decisions and unpleasant experiences.

But removing one risk factor (the ability to make an unwise choice) might result in the creation of another risk (lack of skill in decision-making). Negotiation of choices and decision-making are skills that we have all had to learn, and taking risks and making mistakes can assist us to become 'self-empowered'. Hollomotz concluded that this manipulation of choices about daily activities resulted in '... habitual behaviour... mistaken for active choice and resignation for contentment.' (Hollomotz, 2014, p.247).

Coercion, persuasion and manipulation are all forms of external influence that may interfere with an individual's voluntariness, impeding or diminishing their autonomous choice and action. However, not all influences distort autonomy and control decision-making, and these may be less problematic from a moral viewpoint. Influencing a person's choices through rational persuasion, with the intention of informing their decisions – for example, giving the evidence about the efficacy of a particular intervention or explaining the potential consequences of their actions (even when these may be unpleasant) – appeals to reason rather than emotion. This approach forms part of the procedural requirements of informed consent in health and care, where sufficient appropriate information must be given to enable a person to make a reasoned, autonomous decision.

Having the freedom to make choices and decisions

Being autonomous is most often associated in healthcare with an individual's ability to make their own self-determined choices, having a degree of independence, and the capacity to reason and to reflect on their desires and preferences in their decision-making. It also requires, to some extent, that each person has the freedom to make decisions about, express and act on their personal preferences, desires and goals.

For example, if we said it was in your best interests for you to spend all weekend reading and completing exercises in this book, you might well reply that you have other things planned and, anyway, how do we know what is right for you as you learn best by doing small chunks of study over a period of time. You will base your decision about our suggestion on a range of factors, including your past learning experiences, information guiding your learning (for example advice from tutors and the learning outcomes in a course or module), the immediate relevance of the book to you at this time (for example, an assignment that requires you to say something about your values in practice, due in on Monday), and other demands on your time such as family commitments that impact on your priorities for your weekend. As an autonomous person, you are free to choose whether or not you heed our advice. Equally, in exercising that right to choose, you also have to accept responsibility for your decision.

The same principle applies in health and care. You are generally free to make choices about how you live your life and to make decisions about your own health and wellbeing. Practitioners are limited in what they can do to or for an autonomous person without their consent (with a few exceptions, principally those concerned with temporary lack of competence or capacity to make decisions, e.g. following an accident). However, the notion of freedom of choice in healthcare is not as straightforward as this suggests.

Personal autonomy is generally regarded as distinct from freedom. Freedom is concerned with the ability to act without external or internal constraints and with sufficient resources and power to make your desires effective. Thus, freedom to make healthy choices may depend on having the resources to do so; hence the relevance of strategies to address educational, social and economic determinants of health and tackle inequalities (e.g. RCN, 2012). On the other hand, personal autonomy is concerned with your competence or capacities to be self-governing and the independence and authenticity of the desires that move you to act in the first place.

The concept of freedom on which choice is based is complex and how freedom is defined and interpreted has important implications for social policy and for notions of autonomy. In the context of informed choice and consent in healthcare, freedom in relation to autonomy is principally taken to mean freedom from interference. However, living in a civilised society also requires certain co-operations; inevitably people's preferences and actions may obstruct those of others, and desires will at times conflict such that some of our 'selfish desires' have to be curbed to accommodate the interests of others (Warburton, 2001).

Part of the challenge is about defining the morally permissible limits of individual freedom and choice, what boundaries should be set or specific activities encouraged to achieve certain outcomes, and if and how these should be imposed. These are particularly relevant when considering health policy and strategies which aim to improve population health through encouraging citizens to make healthier and more informed choices and to take responsibility for their own health (DH, 2004a; DH, 2010; Snelling, 2014).

Restrictions on freedom of choice and paternalism

Being autonomous should not be about being self-centred, excessively individualistic or asocial, and consideration must be given to how an individual's freedom to exercise their own autonomy impacts on that of others. You may be justified in not respecting a person's autonomy if their action would result in significant harm to others. This is often attributed to the philosopher John Stuart Mill and referred to in ethics as the Millian 'Harm Principle',

> '… the only purpose for which power can be rightfully exercised over any member
> of a civilized community, against his will, is to prevent harm to others.'
>
> (Mill, 1859, p.6).

For example, as an adult, you are 'free' to choose to drink any amount of alcohol you wish. However, if you then choose to drive while over the legal limit of alcohol we would be justified in trying to stop you because of the risk you would pose to other people, and there would be legal penalties and restrictions of your future freedom through revoking your driving licence or imprisonment. The law which bans smoking in public places restricts freedom of choice and is perhaps more controversial due to its significant infringement of personal liberties. It was argued that individuals who smoke are 'free' to choose to take risks with their own health but should not be able to impose the potential harmful consequences of their choices on others. Legislation which makes it illegal to smoke in cars carrying children, with the aim of protecting under 18s from 'second-hand smoking', is another example. However, if we made attempts to stop you driving or smoking, not on the basis of the risks to others, but because we felt it was in your best interests, we could be deemed to be acting paternalistically.

Questions about the freedom of individual choice also emerge in discussion of resource allocation, prioritisation and rights to healthcare. Should the smoker have free access to healthcare for the treatment of diseases which have a direct causal relationship with smoking? Should the alcohol-dependent individual who develops cirrhosis of the liver be considered for liver transplantation? Personal autonomy, individual choice and freedom, and whether the person was subject to influences, either internal or external, that limited their self-control, as well as the principle of justice and how justice is defined, would be aspects for consideration in any exploration of these moral questions.

Paternalism

Dworkin (1988) was concerned in his account of personal autonomy with the kind of individual freedom that ought to be protected from paternalistic interference. In this way, being autonomous should act as a barrier to unchecked paternalism, and respecting a person's autonomy recognises an individual's freedom to be self-governing and make choices. Paternalism only exists in actions that fail to respect a person's autonomy but are done with the intent of benefiting that person or to prevent them being harmed. Thus, you would be acting paternalistically if the person is at least minimally autonomous and you either:

- prevent a person from acting or force them to act in a particular way, or do something to them without their consent, because it is in their best interests; or
- interfere with their autonomous decision-making by, for example, withholding information, again for their own good.

Whether or not paternalism can ever be justified will depend upon the value placed on acting in someone's best interest versus that of autonomy. Paternalism is more likely to be justified where an individual's autonomy is compromised, although decisions of this kind are highly contentious. For example, should doctors transfuse blood as a life-saving intervention in an emergency situation to an unconscious patient who is a Jehovah's Witness, in spite of their express advance directive that they do not consent to receiving blood? In the past, paternalism was common, with practitioners frequently providing care and interventions without adequate patient involvement in the decision-making process. However, that is now recognised as a controversial approach to practice, and respect for the individual's preferences must be balanced with the degree of risk and harm that may result. You will explore this further in *Chapter 8*: 'Protection from harm and promoting independence'.

Respect for autonomy or paternalism? – the use of electronic tracking devices for people with dementia

Dilemmas associated with balancing autonomy and self-determination against risk and potential harms arise, for example, in the use of electronic tracking devices for monitoring the location of people with dementia who are vulnerable to becoming lost from 'wandering'. 'Wandering' is difficult to define but encompasses a broad range of walking behaviours that can result in a person with dementia leaving his or her dwelling and then becoming 'lost' (Algase *et al.*, 2007). If you review a range of literature in this area (see Activity 6.5) you should be able to identify key ethical concerns and moral arguments for and against the use of such technology with people with dementia. You should consider the arguments from different positions, such as the interests of the person with dementia, those of family and friends and your duties as a healthcare practitioner.

ACTIVITY 6.5

The use of electronic tracking devices for people with dementia

1. Conduct a short literature search using some of the key terms in the title of this activity or access some of the articles listed below:

Algase, D.L. *et al.* (2007) Mapping the maze of terms and definitions in dementia-related wandering. *Aging and Mental Health*, **11(6)**: 686–698.

Bantry White, E. and Montgomery, P. (2014) Electronic tracking for people with dementia: an exploratory study of the ethical issues experienced by carers in making decisions about usage. *Dementia*, **13(2)**: 216–232.

Duggan, S. *et al.* (2008) The impact of early dementia on outdoor life. A 'shrinking world'? *Dementia*, **7(2)**: 191–204.

Niemeijer, A. *et al.* (2015) The experiences of people with dementia and intellectual disabilities with surveillance technologies in residential care. *Nursing Ethics*, **22(3)**: 307–320.

Robinson, L. *et al.* (2007) Balancing rights and risks: conflicting perspectives in the management of wandering in dementia. *Health, Risk and Society*, **9(4)**: 389–406.

2. Read the articles with the main purpose of identifying moral arguments for and against the use of tracking devices with people with dementia. You may want to use the following values or themes as part of your analysis:

   - Respect for persons and dignity
   - Autonomy and freedom
   - Capacity
   - Harms and benefits
   - Risk and prevention of harms
   - Rights
   - Duties and obligations of (and to) others

3. Now read the Alzheimer's Society's position statement *Safer Walking Technology* (Alzheimer's Society, 2013) and refine or add to your arguments alzheimers.org. uk/site/scripts/documents_info.php?documentID=579 (accessed 16 December 2016)

Setting aside the issues in defining 'wandering' and 'getting lost', you may have identified some of the following arguments for and against the use of tracking technology with people with dementia. One perceived benefit could be the continued freedom of movement and supported independence (thus some degree of respect for persons and individual choices). Being able to locate individuals provides reassurances for carers as well as safeguarding people with dementia from potential harms. These harms may be emotional and psychological, such as those arising from intervention to prevent 'wandering' (e.g. locked doors) or actual physical harms, for example, risk from environmental hazards such as long periods in the cold. However, the desire of family, carers and practitioners to protect individuals from harms may be seen as unduly controlling and paternalistic. Benefits may also include supporting the physical activity of walking and enabling some degree of self-determination through freedom of choice to walk where and when they want, on their own without hindrance, but offering secure parameters.

Counter-arguments might include the potential limitations of freedom, deception and the invasion of privacy and breach of confidences through covert surveillance, exacerbated by the stigma through association with electronic tagging used to monitor persistent offenders. This may explain the Alzheimer's Society's preference to refer to this as 'safer walking technology' (Alzheimer's Society, 2013).

Although the use of tracking technology may promote respect for the choices of people with dementia who 'wander', each person may have differing needs, abilities and expectations. Thus, tracking of this kind would be only one strategy to be considered as a part of a person-centred approach to dementia care. This also raises questions as to whether the person with dementia has the competence and capacities to be considered autonomous.

CAPACITY AND COMPETENCE

Anything that limits an individual's personal capacity to weigh up information and make choices will compromise their autonomy. Deciding whether a person has the capacities to be autonomous in decision-making introduces the notion of competence.

ACTIVITY 6.6

Reflection

- What do you understand by the term 'competence'?
- What factors may impact on a service user's or patient's competence?
- Is competence an absolute, all or nothing phenomenon, i.e. is an individual either competent or not competent? Explain your answer.

Competence is not easy to define, and yet it plays a major role in determining whether or not individuals are autonomous, capable of adequate decision-making and should therefore have their own choices about their care respected. While the terms capacity and competence are connected and often used interchangeably, in practice some distinctions can be made. The term 'competence' is often found in philosophical accounts of autonomy, while 'capacity' is formally used in the legal context, specifically the Mental Capacity Act (2005) in English law. 'Capacity' may also be used when referring to a specific task or decision as opposed to a 'global' determination of an individual's competence. However, even this distinction may not be as finely drawn, as you can see in some formal definitions in *Box 6.4*.

BOX — 6.4

Formal definitions of competence

Competence is

'... the capacity to make an explicit, reasoned and intentional choice among alternative courses of action.'

Pellegrino and Thomasma (1988, p.149)

'... Competence, in making medical decisions, is the ability to make a rational decision...[and]... competence is always task-specific.'

Gert, Culver and Clouser (1997, p.137)

Competence determination is of a

'... particular person's capacity to perform a particular decision-making task at a particular time and under specified conditions.'

Buchanan and Brock (1990, p.18)

'... Competency includes various capacities for rational thought, self-control, and freedom from debilitating pathologies, systematic self-deception, and so on.'

Christman (2015, s.1.2)

Beauchamp and Childress (2013, p.115) define competence simply as 'the ability to perform a task'. Think about any task that you have competence to perform. You will recognise that it requires a level of knowledge or information, certain skills and personal and external resources. Remember the first time you rode a bike or drove a car. It would be very unlikely that you had competence from the outset but instead had to learn to perform the task. In this sense, competence should be viewed as being relative to the task to be performed or the decision to be made, so you may be competent to drive a car but not competent to ride a horse.

Welie and Welie (2001, pp.127–8) argue that a more substantive view of competence presupposes a 'coming together' of certain qualities and abilities that result in successfully completing the task or 'getting the job done'. These conditions are:
- Knowing the kind of task to be fulfilled (different tasks require different skills);
- What it means to fulfil the task well (not necessarily excellently but to achieve sufficient results given the circumstances; a threshold concept);
- The abilities or qualities required to do the task well are known; and
- Knowing whether the person charged with undertaking the task has the required qualities or abilities.

However, knowing that a person has the abilities to make sound decisions does not guarantee that they will exercise those abilities in relation to a given task. A person may refuse to behave competently, which may be due to resistance but equally could be because of fear or a breakdown in trust, which then creates problems for judgements of competence in practice.

Bielby (2005, p.358) makes the distinction between agency competence, the general ability or potential to act voluntarily for freely chosen purposes, and task-specific competence, '… the ability of an individual to perform or participate in a specialised activity successfully.' Agency competence is a necessary condition for task-specific competence. Different people will have different competences to different degrees of proficiency due to a range of internal factors (e.g. reasoning, creativity, physical strength) and external factors (relevant information, non-coercive environment). This is why judgements of competence or capacity must be made on an individual basis not attributed to a particular type or group of people.

Competence can also vary over time and be intermittent; you may no longer be able to speak French as fluently as you did in school because you have not practised that learning for some time. It may be refreshed to some degree when you visit France and then diminish again as you do not use the skill in your everyday life. In just the same ways, patients and service users may be competent in some regards but not others, and their competence may change over time depending on a range of circumstances, including their mental or physical state, social determinants or context, or the familiarity or unfamiliarity of a situation, task or decision.

Judgements of competence can be complicated by the need to distinguish between conditions that result in chronic deterioration of intellect, language or memory, such as severe dementia, and those that lead to temporary, reversible states, such as the effects of transient ischaemic attacks. The risk here is that generalised judgements of incompetence may be made inappropriately that exclude the person from all forms of decision-making, now and in the future (Beauchamp and Childress, 2013).

From these accounts and definitions, competence relates to abilities that may be task-specific, although competence in formal definitions of personal autonomy may also be used in a global sense. For example, addicted smokers are autonomous persons in a general sense but may lack competence and be unable to control their behaviour in this one aspect of their lives despite a strong desire to stop smoking.

Standards of competence in making health and care decisions often focus on an individual's capacities to make choices and are closely associated with the internal qualities of being autonomous. This requires the person to be able to:
* understand and process information;
* reason and deliberate and reflect on preferences;
* make a judgement about the information in light of their personal values and goals;
* recognise options and appreciate the significance and meaning of different options and their potential consequences;
* intend a particular outcome or consequences;
* communicate their intentions and wishes, and
* be free from distorting influences, particularly those internal to the individual, such as impaired memory, addiction and some forms of mental illness.

The competence of patients and service users in healthcare is normally judged against their capacity or ability to understand an intervention or task, to deliberate on its risks and benefits and to make a decision in light of these deliberations (Beauchamp and Childress, 2013, p.117). Due to the legal and medical presumption that adults are competent and should be treated as such unless proven otherwise, Beauchamp and Childress (2013, p.118) present a range of inabilities that may be used to distinguish incompetence. These cluster according to three kinds of ability, with the 'ability to state a preference' being the weakest standard (see *Table 6.1*).

Table 6.1 *Inabilities used to judge incompetence*

Type of ability or skill	Inabilities used to judge incompetence
Ability to state a preference (an elementary standard)	• Inability to express or communicate a preference or choice
Abilities to understand information and to appreciate one's situation	• Inability to understand one's situation and its consequences • Inability to understand relevant information
Abilities to reason about a consequential life decision	• Inability to give a reason • Inability to give a rational reason (although some supporting reasons may be given) • Inability to give risk-/benefit-related reasons (although some supporting reasons may be given) • Inability to reach a reasonable decision (as judged by a reasonable person)

Adapted from Beauchamp and Childress, 2013, p.118.

You will no doubt see a range of strategies used to judge competence of patients and service users in your practice that will inevitably impact on the degree to which they are deemed to be autonomous and how far their wishes and preferences are acknowledged and respected. An increasing gravity of the consequences of their decision may demand a higher level of competence.

An individual's capacity in autonomous decision-making may be affected by mental illness, learning disability, dementia, brain injury or other disease processes. Capacity may also be affected temporarily by, for example, fear, pain or confusion. However, you should never assume that what affects one person will lead to the same level of incapacity in another. Likewise, care must be taken when individuals make what seems to be an irrational decision; it is important to see the situation through the patient's eyes and from their value position. What is right for you is not necessarily what is right for another and it may be a fine line between competence and incompetence when people choose to make unreasonable, eccentric or unwise decisions.

Legislation relating to capacity in care practice

The values, principles and duties surrounding capacity in health and care are reinforced by the legal standards expressed in the Mental Capacity Act (MCA)(2005) enforced in April 2007. The Act intends

> '... to be enabling and supportive of people who lack capacity, not restricting or controlling of their lives. It aims to protect people who lack capacity to make particular decisions, but also to maximise their ability to make decisions, or to participate in decision-making, as far as they are able to do so.'
>
> (Department for Constitutional Affairs (DCA), 2007, p.19)

The Mental Capacity Act (2005) aims to place individuals at the heart of the decision-making process, to facilitate and support their participation wherever possible and to ensure that any decisions that have to be made on their behalf are done so in their best interests. It also provides the framework for people to plan ahead for a time when they might lack capacity to make decisions for themselves in the future. It sets out five 'statutory principles' that support the legal requirements in the Act (see *Box 6.5*) which are in turn underpinned by a number of moral values.

Principles 1 to 3 of the Act reflect the value of respect for persons and the presumption of personal autonomy unless lack of capacity is established. Principle 2 also implies a duty to support or enable autonomous decision-making wherever possible. Principle 4 involves the value of beneficence with concern for acting in a person's best interests. Principle 5 makes reference to the least restrictive course of action that impacts on a person's rights and freedoms and uses human rights as constraints on the interpretation and implementation of the 'best interests' principle. Thus, compliance with the Act

BOX — 6.5

Section 1 of the Mental Capacity Act

The five statutory principles are:

1. A person must be assumed to have capacity unless it is established that they lack capacity.

2. A person is not to be treated as unable to make a decision unless all practicable steps to help him to do so have been taken without success.

3. A person is not to be treated as unable to make a decision merely because he makes an unwise decision.

4. An act done, or decision made, under this Act for or on behalf of a person who lacks capacity must be done, or made, in his best interests.

5. Before the act is done, or the decision is made, regard must be had to whether the purpose for which it is needed can be as effectively achieved in a way that is less restrictive of the person's rights and freedom of action.

'Following the principles and applying them to the Act's framework for decision-making will help to ensure not only that appropriate action is taken in individual cases, but also to point the way to solutions in difficult or uncertain situations.

A person's capacity (or lack of capacity) refers specifically to their capacity to make a particular decision at the time it needs to be made.'

Source: *Mental Capacity Act 2005 Code of Practice* (DCA, 2007, p.19).

should protect persons who lack capacity from forms of abuse, threat and coercion, exploitation, disrespect or unwarranted intrusions on their privacy and liberty (Mackenzie and Rogers, 2013, p.38).

Throughout the *Mental Capacity Act 2005 Code of Practice* (DCA, 2007), capacity is defined simply as the ability to make a decision, which includes decisions that affect daily life, e.g. deciding when to get up or what to wear, as well as more serious or significant decisions that may have legal consequences for themselves or others, e.g. deciding whether to give consent for medical treatment or making a will. The Act views capacity as both decision- and time-specific, and assessment must only examine a person's capacity to make a particular decision at the specific time it needs to be made. It does not matter if the incapacity is temporary, or the person retains the capacity to make other decisions, or if the person's capacity fluctuates. This means an individual may lack capacity to make a decision at one time but have the capacity to make the same decision at another. Similarly, an individual may be unable to make a decision regarding a certain matter but at the same time have capacity to make a decision about something else.

This specificity in assessing capacity allows for the potential intermittent nature of personal autonomy and fluctuations in agency and task-specific competence described earlier.

It also supports the least restrictive approach to judgements of capacity (see *Box 6.6*). In this way, the Act aims to promote the autonomy of vulnerable persons whenever possible and to provide protection for those individuals who lack capacity or whose capacity may be partially compromised who are vulnerable to harms and to paternalistic intervention by others. This means that practitioners and carers must be aware of potential influences on and changes in an individual's capacity and the need for capacity to be re-assessed (HMSO, 2014). Also, from the principle of fairness and treating people equally, a person's capacity must not be judged simply on the basis of their age, appearance, condition or an aspect of their behaviour. You need to be culturally sensitive (Herissone-Kelly, 2010) and mindful that considerable effort and support is needed to enable some patients with minimal levels of capacity to make autonomous decisions if you are to guard against unwarranted paternalism and disrespect (Mackenzie and Rogers, 2013).

BOX — 6.6

Assessing capacity

Anyone assessing someone's capacity to make a decision for themselves should use the two-stage test of capacity used within the Mental Capacity Act 2005 (DCA, 2007, p.44–5):

Stage 1: Does the person have an impairment of, or a disturbance in the functioning of, their mind or brain?

This could include conditions associated with some forms of mental illness, dementia, significant learning disabilities, long-term effects of brain damage, physical or medical conditions that cause confusion, drowsiness or loss of consciousness and symptoms of alcohol or drug use.

Stage 2: Does the impairment or disturbance mean that the person is unable to make a specific decision when they need to?

Assessing ability to make a decision (DCA, 2007, p.41)

- Does the person have a general understanding of what decision they need to make and why they need to make it?
- Does the person have a general understanding of the likely consequences of making, or not making, this decision?
- Is the person able to understand, retain, use and weigh up the information relevant to this decision?
- Can the person communicate their decision (by talking, using sign language or any other means)? Would the services of a professional (such as a speech and language therapist) be helpful?

Assessing capacity to make more complex or serious decisions

- Is there a need for a more thorough assessment (perhaps by involving a doctor or other professional expert)?

Adapted from the *Mental Capacity Act 2005 Code of Practice* (DCA, 2007, pp.41–5).

The *Mental Capacity Act 2005 Code of Practice* (DCA, 2007) identifies those people who have a formal duty to observe the Code, including professionals and paid carers, and how the statutory principles should be applied in practice. It also provides guidance for less formal carers, family and friends. You should read the *Mental Capacity Act 2005 Code of Practice*, as it provides a wealth of practice examples that will challenge and consolidate your understanding of the issues associated with the competence of patients and service users and their participation in care decisions.

According to an inquiry into the implementation of the MCA (House of Lords Select Committee on the Mental Capacity Act 2005, 2014), legislation alone may be insufficient in changing attitudes and behaviours in practice. However, the notion of capacity and competence in personal autonomy is complex and supporting patient autonomy is not only about big, life-changing decisions. If one of the aims of the MCA is protection of vulnerable adults from unwarranted paternalism, then instances of everyday care should also be subject to the principles in the Act. However, it is the attitudes of carers and their understanding of the values of respect for persons, dignity and autonomy that are crucial to providing, supporting and enhancing opportunities for autonomous choice and decision-making, particularly for those with, or at risk of, diminished capacity.

A DUTY OF RESPECT FOR AUTONOMY

From our earlier discussion of respect for persons and the value placed on being autonomous, it follows that respect for autonomy is one of the fundamental principles that should guide your interactions with patients and service users and the care that you provide. Respecting autonomy in practice means, at the very least, that you acknowledge a person's:

> '... rights to hold views, to make choices, and to take actions based on their values and beliefs. Such respect involves respectful action, not merely a respectful attitude. It also requires more than non-interference in others' personal affairs.'
> (Beauchamp and Childress, 2013, pp.106–7)

In order to respect the autonomy of patients and service users you will need to:
- listen and communicate effectively;
- help to develop or maintain their capacities for autonomous choice;
- provide relevant information at an appropriate level of understanding and in a medium suitable for the patient or service user;
- support the development of necessary skills, including cognitive abilities;
- enable individuals to make decisions voluntarily and freely;
- help to dispel fears and other conditions that could impede autonomous decision-making and action;

- ensure the environment is conducive to their decision-making;
- accept their choices and respect their decisions, including decisions to refuse or withdraw from treatment or intervention, whatever the outcome; and
- acknowledge the value and decision-making rights of autonomous persons.

Respecting autonomy is not just about agreeing with the wishes of others. If you view autonomy as a quality, respect may also involve the creation or increase of their autonomy and using strategies to enable individuals to make reasoned choices. It is not about simply saying 'over to you' when there are difficult decisions to be made. Autonomy should be thought of more broadly, and concern for service user and patient welfare is, in itself, a central part of autonomy creation. Without advice, support and education, an individual may have little or no autonomy to exercise (Seedhouse, 2009, pp.148–50).

Advocacy (ensuring the voice of the patient or service user is heard and seeing the world from the individual's perspective) and empowerment (supporting the development of an individual's skills and self-confidence) are valuable enabling strategies that can enhance respect for the individual and their autonomy in their care decisions. The increasing emphasis on individual choice and the ideology of recovery in mental health practice (which assesses health improvement through an individual's own experience, develops resilience and recovery of hope and ambition for living full and purposeful lives, and achieving choice and control for individuals and their families) also reflects the values of respect, dignity and autonomy. There is insufficient scope in this book to do full justice to these concepts and you are advised to follow up this chapter by reading about these specific areas of work.

The principle of respect for autonomy also supports other moral rules for practice, such as respecting privacy (addressed in *Chapter 4*) and truth-telling and protecting confidentiality which we turn to in *Chapter 7* in relation to the value of trust and trustworthiness. Informed consent provides one of the clearest applications of respect for autonomy in practice.

INFORMED CONSENT

Consent is a fundamental moral and legal concept in health and care practice and is clearly grounded in the principle of respect for persons and their autonomy. Consent is an expression of a person's right to autonomy, and consent should be sought not only before any medical or healthcare intervention but also in providing fundamental care and meeting personal care needs. Consent acts as a legal defence for practitioners. It is unlawful to touch another person without their agreement and you may be liable in both civil and criminal law if you do so, resulting in claims of negligence, trespass to the person and battery. Thus consent makes what would otherwise be unlawful lawful and there are few exceptions to the duty of consent; lack of capacity to make decisions is the most significant (Taylor, 2013).

On first sight, the legal role of consent could be viewed as being concerned with the protection of healthcare practitioners. However, the moral obligation is primarily to protect patients and service users, their right to respect for their autonomy and their status as autonomous individuals who have interests in being self-determining and remaining in control of their own lives (Farsides, 2013, p.151). Moral values and justifications for consent inevitably underpin much of what is understood from a legal or professional perspective.

What is the value associated with informed consent?

Consent can be simply defined as giving someone permission to do something that they would not otherwise have the right to do. In health and care, consent is usually referred to as informed consent, which is taken to mean 'informed, voluntary and decisionally-capacitated consent' (Eyal, 2012, p.2). This reflects the right of individuals to give or to refuse consent as a fundamental way of expressing and exercising their autonomy and in protecting their bodily integrity. It also protects autonomous individuals from particular harms.

Participating in the consent process can further enhance an individual's personal autonomy through their acquisition of new knowledge, utilising decision-making skills, developing confidence and taking responsibility for decisions. In this way, personal autonomy is both a prerequisite for consent as well as a product of consent (Farsides, 2013). Giving consent to care, interventions and treatment is also the ultimate expression of trust in another.

> 'Informed consent is one hallmark of trust between strangers. For example, when I understand a pension plan, a mortgage, or complex medical procedures, and am free to choose or refuse, I express my trust by giving informed consent. We give informed consent in face-to-face transactions too, though we barely notice it. We buy apples in the market, we exchange addresses with acquaintances, we sit down for a haircut. It sounds pompous to speak of these daily transactions as based on informed consent: yet in each we assume that the other party is neither deceiving nor coercing. We withdraw our trust very fast if we are sold rotten apples, or deliberately given a false address, or forcibly subjected to a Mohican haircut.'
>
> (O'Neill, 2002c, p.1)

As informed consent is an expression of having trust in another, a person must already trust you in order to give their consent. They may rely on you to provide accurate and reliable information and on 'experts' to help them to assess the quality and effectiveness of interventions, but they must already trust these people not to deceive or have bad intentions. How they have arrived at this trust relates to their various experiences of the care relationship, such as whether or not their confidences have been respected.

Informed consent is therefore important for several reasons:
- From the value attributed to respect for persons, being autonomous and respect for an individual's autonomy
- Having to obtain consent offers protection of the individual from harm (or at least unwarranted or uninvited harms), including to their bodily integrity and privacy
- From a principle of concern for their welfare and best interests
- It fosters trust and confidence
- Promotes patient and service user responsibility for their health and wellbeing
- Protection of the practitioner
- It is required by law.

The value of respect for persons and respect for their autonomy through consent

Respect for persons is fundamental in health and care and people should be supported and enabled to be self-determining. Being autonomous also entails that people will take control of and be responsible for their own lives. Thus consent is essential to any duty of respect for autonomy and expects individuals to make their own choices regarding what does or does not happen to them. All of the factors already discussed that are required to be autonomous and those that can prevent people from being autonomous apply to the consent process.

Gillon's (1986, p.115) definition captures the essential moral features of consent:

> 'a voluntary uncoerced decision, made by a sufficiently competent or autonomous person on the basis of adequate information and deliberation, to accept rather than reject some proposed course of action which will affect him or her.'

You should recognise key components in this definition arising from the value of autonomy and the conditions necessary to be autonomous. The person giving consent should be 'sufficiently competent' (have mental capacity) and the decision that is the outcome of the consent process should be a 'voluntary, deliberate and uncoerced choice' based on consideration of 'adequate information' (see *Box 6.7*).

Informed consent places demands on practitioners to provide sufficient and appropriate information and to ensure that they do or say nothing that might coerce or manipulate the patient or restrict their voluntariness in decision-making. Practitioners should allow time and space, wherever possible, for individuals to assimilate the information provided and to deliberate on their options in order to reach a decision that is their own to consent or to withhold consent. Autonomy is less likely to be compromised if the environment and the way in which consent is discussed aim to enable the person to feel as much at ease as possible rather than embarrassed, intimidated or distressed (Farsides, 2005).

BOX — **6.7**

The general requirements for informed consent and necessary conditions for autonomy

- The person has the competence to understand, retain and weigh up information and express their preferences and make choices.

- Freedom from overwhelming influences or interferences (such as manipulation and coercion); voluntariness or making voluntary choices and decisions (this includes the freedom to refuse or withhold consent).

- Disclosure of sufficient and accurate information and having understanding of this information as a basis for their decision-making (includes time to deliberate on options).

- Adequate information normally entails giving all the information relevant to their decision (except where it may cause serious harm). Includes:

  o an explanation of what is to happen, e.g. the intervention, type of care

  o the relevant facts and probabilities of success or failure associated with options and the benefits and potential harms

  o a requirement on the part of the practitioner or carer to acquire sufficient information from the patient, in order to know their goals, what information is needed and what type of help or care the patient wants.

- Consent also requires that a decision is made.

Whenever possible, it is important to treat obtaining consent as a process, not a one-off event. Patients and service users often need time to think through the options and consequences of their decisions, ask questions, check their understanding and seek further information before arriving at their final decision. The competent adult is also free to change their mind and withdraw consent at any time. If there is any doubt, you should always check that they still consent to you caring for or treating them.

Concern for their welfare and best interests

If in seeking consent we are concerned with enabling the individual to be self-determining, we should also assume that the competent person will be the best judge of what is in their best interests. Thus, informed consent may act both as a protection from paternalism as well as promoting the welfare and best interests of the patient.

Although practitioners may have knowledge and expertise they can use to inform and offer the 'best' clinical decision regarding treatment or intervention, they may not be the best judge of other factors that matter equally or more importantly to the patient or service user, such as those arising from their particular cultural or religious background. You must be careful not to judge the person's decisions according to what you would want for yourself or to manipulate their decision in order to ensure that it concurs with what you determine to be in their best interests. However, you may help them understand that certain courses of action may result in 'better' or different outcomes (if this is the case) which then may inform their determination of what is the best decision for them. The requirement to provide adequate information means that this should also be balanced, i.e. both the potential harms and benefits are identified. 'Acquiescence when a patient does not know what the intervention entails, or is unaware that he or she can refuse, is not "consent".' (BMA, 2009b, p.7)

Individuals who are fully informed about and involved in the decisions about their care may also be more likely to trust the practitioner and participate in their care, thus contributing to their overall wellbeing. (See *Box 6.8* for guidance on helping someone make a decision for themselves.)

BOX 6.8

Helping someone make a decision for themselves

To do this, check the following points:

Providing relevant information

- Does the person have all the relevant information they need to make a particular decision?
- If they have a choice, have they been given information on all the alternatives?

Communicating in an appropriate way

Could information be explained or presented in a way that is easier for the person to understand (for example, by using simple language or visual aids)?

- Have different methods of communication been explored if required, including non-verbal communication?
- Could anyone else help with communication (for example, a family member, support worker, interpreter, speech and language therapist or advocate)?

Making the person feel at ease

- Are there particular times of day when the person's understanding is better?
- Are there particular locations where they may feel more at ease?
- Could the decision be put off to see whether the person can make the decision at a later time when circumstances are right for them?

Supporting the person

- Can anyone else help or support the person to make choices or express a view?

Source: *Mental Capacity Act 2005 Code of Practice* (DCA, 2007, p.29).

What is required by law?

There is no English statute setting out the principles of consent, other than those related to mental capacity (Mental Capacity Act, 2005, c.9). The requirement of consent is based principally in the right of competent individuals to self-determination and in the common law (case law) which establishes the offence of battery if a person is touched without their valid consent. The tort of negligence may also apply, for example, if there was a breach of duty of care and harms resulted because the consent process was insufficiently informed.

Consent may be either explicit or implied:

*   *Explicit consent* – usually given orally or in writing and conveys a clear indication of the individual's preference or choice related to a specific intervention or aspect of care. The decision should be made freely and voluntarily in light of knowledge of the available options and their consequences. Written consent is normally the responsibility of the professional providing the treatment or intervention. It is more than just a signature on a form and should be the outcome of open dialogue and communication between professional and patient. Oral consent for less risky interventions is common practice but harder to evidence.
*   *Implied consent* – where agreement to a course of action has been demonstrated by a person's behaviour, e.g. when they willingly offer their arm for blood pressure monitoring. Implied consent is not a lesser form of consent and it cannot be assumed. It should still meet the necessary conditions, such that you are confident that the individual genuinely knows and understands what is being proposed on the basis of adequate information.

Both forms of consent are equally relevant in law, although it is easier to validate explicit consent, particularly if written. Failure to gain proper consent for an intervention that later causes the patient or service user harm may be used in claims of negligence. Poor consent processes may also result in complaints, either through employers or professional bodies or both. Written explicit consent is usually supported by documentation, such as that provided by the Department of Health (DH, 2009). However, much of the consent you will obtain for everyday care interventions will be either verbal or implied. Thus, it is particularly important that you maintain accurate records of care and document where explicit verbal consent has been given and the process used to establish consent prior to care interventions.

The Mental Capacity Act (2005, c.9) and its *Code of Practice* (DCA, 2007) are also essential sources when determining a person's capacity to give or withhold their consent. Other good sources of professional guidance include the British Medical Association Consent Tool Kit (BMA, 2009b), professional codes of conduct (e.g. NMC, 2015) and the Department of Health *Reference Guide to Consent for Examination or Treatment,*

2ⁿᵈ ed (DH, 2009b) available at www.gov.uk/government/publications/reference-guide-to-consent-for-examination-or-treatment-second-edition (accessed 16 December 2016). This includes guidance on meeting the specific needs of a range of individuals in the consent process, including children and young people, older people and people with learning disabilities.

Completing the activity in *Case study 6.1* should help you to consolidate your thoughts on the principle of respect for autonomy and its relationship with the duty of informed consent. You will also start to consider the rights and wrongs of truth-telling and deception and to think about the importance of consent as an expression of trust in the healthcare relationship.

CASE STUDY 6.1

Covert administration of medication

Mary is a 79-year-old resident in the care home where you work as a care assistant. She has asthma that is generally well controlled. Recently, she developed a chest infection and has been prescribed two courses of antibiotics. However, although she recognises that the antibiotics are for her benefit, they are making her feel particularly unwell, with constant nausea and diarrhoea. When you and the care home manager take her the next dose of antibiotic, she refuses to take it saying, 'I can't take any more of these horrible things. Surely I have had enough of them by now. My family are visiting tomorrow, bringing my new grandson, and I don't want to feel lousy.' You both try to encourage her to take the tablets but she continues to refuse them.

The manager is concerned; she knows the importance of giving the antibiotics at the prescribed intervals and that Mary should finish the course of medication, particularly as her asthma has been less well controlled since having the chest infection. She asks you to conceal the medication in her food; she feels that it is more important that she has the antibiotics as she is fearful that she will develop pneumonia.

- What should you do?

Giving medication to a patient or service user normally requires their consent.

- Why should you obtain consent?
- What are the moral justifications for informed consent?
- Can Mary refuse the medication as part of the consent process?
- Are there any instances where consent would not be required?
- Is deception through the covert administration of medication justified in this case? Explain your answers.

The covert administration of medication is a controversial issue, particularly in cases where individuals are autonomous and have the capacity to make their own choices about what is right for them. There is no reason from the information given here to question Mary's capacity using the criteria in the Mental Capacity Act 2005. She has made a decision and has given a perfectly rational reason for it, based on her knowledge and experience of the effects of the medication. On this basis, she has the right to refuse the medication even though her refusal may not concur with what others believe is in her best interests. You must respect her refusal just as much as you would her consent (see *Box 6.9*).

In disguising the medication in Mary's food or drink, she is being led to believe that she is not receiving medication, when in fact she is. This is an obvious case of deception which interferes with her freedom and voluntariness in decision-making. The manager's motive in doing so appears well intentioned, depending on weighing the harms associated with her chest infection against the discomfort and distress caused

---

BOX 6.9

The consent process – translating theory into practice

Translating a theoretical commitment to respect for autonomy into practice in the consent process in care requires the practitioner to develop certain skills and accept responsibility to action them. These include:

- assessing autonomy, competence and voluntariness
- respecting autonomy where it is present
- creating and enhancing autonomy where it is lacking, and promoting best interests and wellbeing
- being involved in providing evidence-based information and establishing the extent of the patient's understanding, reflection and deliberation (this will often not occur in a direct way but be evident through passing comments, non-verbal signs and expression of anxieties and misinterpretations)
- communicating effectively with the patient and their family – developing understanding of the patient as an individual and their social context, listening and establishing their expectations and preferences, providing information in a variety of forms
- balancing being 'non-directive' (generally accepted as not interfering with autonomy) with being seen to be 'unsupportive' (for example in answering the question, 'What would you do?')
- developing cultural literacy – understanding the cultural context, the beliefs, values and practices of different groups
- fostering supportive care relationship and environment – helping individuals to engage with the consent process, ensuring the patient's voice is heard including when this conflicts with family and other professionals, being non-judgemental and willing to convey the view of the individual even when this contradicts your own.

Adapted from Farsides, 2013, pp.147–9.

---

by the side-effects of the antibiotics. On balance, the better course of action would be to ask her General Practitioner if the antibiotics could be changed to avoid the side-effects.

As the care assistant you have been put in a difficult position; if you do as you have been asked, you would be held responsible for covertly administering the medication, although the manager would be accountable for her instruction. If Mary realises what you have both done, this could cause her distress and could easily destroy any relationship of trust you have with her and subsequently impact on her health and welfare. If she tells other residents, they too may become suspicious, lose faith and trust in the carers' actions and feel a sense of abandonment by those who should be caring for them.

AN ALTERNATIVE VIEW OF AUTONOMY – RELATIONAL AUTONOMY

Before we end this chapter, it is worth introducing an alternative view of autonomy that is rising in popularity in healthcare literature; that of relational autonomy. Viewing autonomy through a relational lens challenges the common procedural accounts and brings additional elements to our understanding of respect for autonomy that sit well with a philosophy of value-based care.

Common understandings of autonomy in healthcare have been heavily influenced by a liberal view of autonomy; self-governance and self-determination; self-rule and self-mastery, being true to oneself and being one's own person. This approach is clearly evident in the processes of informed choice and consent. These accounts rely principally on a notion of autonomy that sees persons as individuals with limited reference to their connections with other people, groups, institutions or traditions with whom or in which they may live or act. Hence the expectations of non-interference and voluntariness in respect for autonomy and consent.

This alignment of autonomy with the ideal of individualism has been criticised as presenting people as atomistic, self-reliant and self-sufficient (Code, 1991). This is seen as overvaluing culturally 'masculine traits' such as independence, impartiality and reason and undervalues culturally 'feminine traits' such as interdependence, connection, emotion and partiality (Mackenzie and Stoljar, 2000).

For many people, making decisions about their own health and care is not simply a question of 'what is best for me alone', but also concerns the impact of their decisions on others with whom they have relationships, responsibilities and concerns. For example, think about cases where women refuse life-saving cancer treatment during pregnancy to 'protect' their baby or a relative who volunteers to be a 'living donor' for a kidney transplant.

Relational autonomy has no single definition and encompasses a range of approaches to understanding autonomy (e.g. Sherwin, 1998; Mackenzie and Stoljar, 2000) but generally accepts:

- the complex nature of autonomous persons and their rich social, interpersonal and historical contexts which impact not only on their identity and self-concept but also their capacities for autonomy
- that social relationships and human community are central to the realisation of autonomy
- sensitivity to our social embeddedness, our interdependence, our mutual support and to the relations of care.

The intention is not to reject fully the notion of individual autonomy but to reframe it in ways that embrace a richer account of autonomous agency and a social conception of the self. This takes account of what it is to be a free, self-governing agent who is also socially constituted and defines an individual's basic values and commitments from a position of interpersonal relationships and mutual dependencies (Christman, 2004, p.143).

BOX **6.10**

Relational autonomy

- Autonomous agency takes account of the interconnectedness between self-concept and the complexities of the social and historical contexts in which the self is developed and situated.
- Analyses the contribution of oppressive social relationships to our understanding of autonomy.
- Emphasises the social and psychological differentiation of human agency.
- Highlights the importance of features such as memory, imagination and emotional dispositions and attitudes.
- Autonomous agents are seen as emotional, embodied, desiring, creative and feeling as well as rational beings.

Source: Mackenzie and Stoljar, 2000, p.21.

Implications for practice

Understanding autonomy relationally encourages practitioners to:

- acknowledge the influence of the socialisation process on development of autonomy competencies
- take account of the network of relationships that influence an individual's efforts to be self-determining, responsible agents

- understand the wider social dynamics, structures and influences on a person's autonomous decision-making
- respond sensitively to the patient's own understandings and experiences of health, wellbeing and ill health
- deliberately support the person's decision-making within the many relationships that they value and which inform their lives rather than as isolated, rational individuals
- make explicit the influence of the person's broader network of social and familial relations that impact on their decision-making, whilst recognising the potential of relationships to both enhance and undermine autonomy
- use their power and influence to restore and strengthen autonomy competencies
- appreciate the continuous nature of relational autonomy rather than seeing healthcare choices as 'one-off events'
- make sense of the apparent altruism some people show in making choices.

Thus, taking relational autonomy into account requires:
- effective interpersonal communication – not only providing accurate, objective, relevant and culturally appropriate information but also establishing and considering each person's personal values, goals and beliefs
- commitment to providing culturally sensitive care
- displaying moral integrity and competence in addressing patients' needs
- developing reciprocal trust and being able to accept and trust people to know what is best for themselves, where trust forms the bridge between a person's autonomous choices which may conflict with a practitioner's view of their best interests
- acknowledging that responsibility becomes a shared component of a relational model of informed choice.

Commitment to relational autonomy works best through a model of sustained person-centred care. The value of a relational approach in understanding autonomy is evident in informing practitioner relationships and advocacy in healthcare (Entwistle *et al.*, 2010; Cole, Wellard and Mummery, 2014), in accounts of the woman-centred philosophy of midwifery (Kirkham, 2010), in approaches to palliative care (Wilson *et al.*, 2014), in person-centred dementia care (Kitwood, 1997; Brooker, 2003; Brooker and Latham, 2015) and is emerging as an alternative view to public health ethics (Owens and Cribb, 2013).

CONCLUSION

One of the dilemmas for practitioners caring for others will always be how to reconcile concern for welfare with respect for autonomy when the two come into conflict. Independence and the ability to live life according to one's own preferences, beliefs and choices are important values in maintaining a good quality of life. What is important is that you do not take for granted or make assumptions about people's ability or inability to be autonomous or deny them the respect that humanity deserves.

This chapter has focused on the value of autonomy and demonstrates that respect for autonomy is fundamental to healthcare practice. Being respected, having our views taken seriously, being able to express our individuality and being able to make, and act on our own choices and decisions are important features of our everyday lives. It is these things that give us a sense of worth and a sense of self. It is therefore essential that you develop your practice in ways that show proper respect for the autonomy of patients and service users. The activities in the chapter have provided you with the opportunity to examine your own approach to care and to think about strategies that would enable you to provide opportunities to support those in your care to be autonomous.

CHAPTER SUMMARY

Four key points to take away from Chapter 6:

- The value of autonomy is fundamental to care practice.
- Respect for autonomy contributes to our sense of worth and a sense of self.
- 'Being autonomous' requires a number of conditions, including the capacity to determine your own goals, make choices and being free to act on the basis of your decisions.
- Respect for autonomy also includes developing care strategies to support and enable others to be autonomous.

FURTHER READING

Beauchamp, T. and Childress, J. (2013) *Principles of Biomedical Ethics*, 7th ed. New York: Oxford University Press, Chapter 4, pp.101–49.

Department for Constitutional Affairs (2007) *Mental Capacity Act 2005. Code of Practice*. Crown Copyright. London: The Stationery Office.

Farsides, B. (2013) 'Consent and the Capable Adult Patient. B: An Ethical Perspective – Consent and Patient Autonomy' in Tingle, J. and Cribb, A. (eds) *Nursing Law and Ethics*, 4th ed. Oxford: Blackwell-Wiley, Ch. 7, pp.151–65.

07

TRUST, CONFIDENTIALITY AND TRUTH-TELLING

LEARNING OUTCOMES:

In this chapter you will:

- Explore the value of trust and trustworthiness and recognise the importance of trust in the practitioner–patient/service user relationship

- Define the origins of a duty of confidentiality and discuss the justifications for such a duty

- Examine the possible exceptions to the obligation of confidentiality

- Explore the value of honesty and truth-telling in the context of health and care

- Reflect on care strategies that promote trust and trustworthiness in practice.

INTRODUCTION

One of the values that seemed to lose prominence in healthcare ethics with the rise in emphasis placed on respect for autonomy, yet is fundamental to health and care practice, is that of trust or trustworthiness. It can be argued that 'trust' is at the very heart of the care relationship. It is difficult, if not impossible, to form a good therapeutic relationship without trust between the individuals involved (Dinç and Gastmans, 2013). Service users and patients need to be confident that they can trust the practitioners delivering their care to be concerned for their wellbeing. We seek guidance, support and care when we have health or social care needs and trust that those caring for us will be knowledgeable and skilled in their particular area of practice. However, this can mean that the relationship between the practitioner and those receiving care can be an unequal one, in which the practitioner may hold at least some power over the service user or patient simply because of their role and expertise. Much work has been done in recent years to shift this balance of power and to enable patients and service users to retain control and have a voice in decision-making at individual, community, service and policy levels. Hence, respect for autonomy has emerged as a primary guiding principle, with the notion of trust becoming associated with more paternalistic approaches to care.

Yet even in a model of care that gives primacy to patient autonomy, trust is still an essential characteristic in the care relationship. You have already seen that to be autonomous requires a number of attributes, such as adequate knowledge and information, and ability for critical reflection and decision-making that may need to be fostered and supported through the therapeutic relationship. Thus, service users, patients and carers must still have confidence in, and be able to rely on, the practitioner to provide not only relevant information, guidance and support but also to intervene and act appropriately with our interests in mind when required.

We place trust in others every day of our lives; we trust people to do what they say they will do, to play by the rules and to behave reasonably (O'Neill, 2002a). If we didn't, living in society would be extremely difficult. Being able to trust makes our life in a social context easier and worthwhile and enables us to fulfil activities alongside others that we could not achieve on our own. We trust our friends to keep secrets, the person to whom we lend money to return it, nurseries to care for our children, other citizens to abide by agreed rules and laws of society.

This chapter explores the value of trust and trustworthiness in health and social care and aims to assist you to reflect on your development as a trustworthy practitioner, paying particular attention to the notions of confidentiality and truthfulness.

WHAT ARE TRUST AND TRUSTWORTHINESS?

'… Each of us and every profession and every institution needs trust. We need it because we have to be able to rely on others acting as they say that they will, and because we need others to accept that we will act as we say we will. The sociologist Niklas Luhman was right that "A complete absence of trust would prevent [one] even getting up in the morning".'

(O'Neill, 2002a, p.1)

'… And when we place trust we don't simply assume that others are reliable and predictable, as we assume that the sun rises reliably, and the milk goes off predictably. When we trust we know – at least when we are no longer small children – that we could be disappointed. Sometimes we place trust in spite of past disappointment, or without much evidence of reliability. To withdraw trust after a single lapse, as if we were rejecting a scientific theory in the face of decisive evidence, would often seem suspicious, even paranoid. All trust risks disappointment. The risk of disappointment, even of betrayal cannot be written out of our lives. Samuel Johnson put it this way: "It is happier to be sometimes cheated than not to trust". Trust is needed not because everything is wholly predictable, or wholly guaranteed, but on the contrary because life has to be led without guarantees.'

(O'Neill, 2002b, p.1)

Trust is an important concept in all of the human services and caring disciplines but although trust is an everyday concept, it may be defined and utilised in a number of ways. Trust can be used to describe the foundation and nature of therapeutic relationships, as a personal attribute or as a quality of interprofessional relationships. It can also be seen as a need, or as a duty or obligation of one person or persons to another and we may place trust in individuals, groups, institutions or societies. Trust is an attitude we have towards other people who we hope will be trustworthy, whereas trustworthiness is a property or characteristic of individuals which can be described in moral terms and as a virtue.

Trust is a word used in everyday language, and it can be viewed from a number of perspectives. A standard account of trust presumes that trust between individuals depends on either direct information or experience of another or indirect knowledge of the individual due to the role they hold. It would be rare to trust people implicitly and completely without any knowledge or experience. It is also important that the trust might extend only to the confines of that role; for example, I might trust a qualified electrician to rewire my home but not to look after my child. Dinç and Gastmans (2013) identify that nurses specifically, and to some extent other care practitioners, are highly trusted even when there is a level of mistrust in the healthcare system. However, these preconceptions are then either reinforced or damaged by the quality of the ensuing personal relationship that is established between the practitioner and the patient. Congruence, or otherwise, between expectations of the relationship and the reality of the actual experience will dictate the effectiveness of the trust relationship.

Putting your trust in another inevitably leads to an expectation that others will be both reliable and dependable, although trusting always involves an element of risk, as there are often no guarantees that the person or institution will live up to the expectations of the individual who has placed their trust. Trust in the health and social care professions has taken some significant knocks over recent years and the centrality of trust has been threatened, as outlined in inquiries such as the Kennedy Report (2001) and Francis Inquiry Report (Francis, 2013). While it cannot be denied that serious and inexcusable harm and suffering occurred in these and similar cases, it is important to remember that such behaviour is not reflective of the vast majority.

Professional bodies and sector skills councils continue to work to promote trust as a primary professional value. It is evident in standards, competency frameworks, policies and guidelines for practice and the value of trustworthiness is reinforced and espoused in all codes of practice. Thus the importance of maintaining, justifying and enhancing the trust placed by individuals in health and care practitioners is taken seriously, whether or not they are professionally registered. Any care relationship is a privileged one; neither practitioners nor individuals in their care have any real choice with whom they form a relationship. They may have little or nothing in common with each other and yet the carer assumes a role in, and has access to, the most personal and intimate aspects of the service user or patient's life. Thus trust is fundamental to the individual's confidence in the practitioner and if trust breaks down at this level it can have detrimental effects both for the patient or service user and for the service as a whole.

With the increasing emphasis on working in partnership with patients and service users to provide optimum care, building a relationship of mutual respect and trust is essential. Establishing a rapport and getting to know the patient as a person is identified as a pre-condition for a good trusting relationship (Belcher, 2009). An individual must feel that the care they receive is specific and tailored to their unique needs. Additionally, being valued, feeling emotionally and physically safe and the availability of and accessibility to those providing care are all prerequisites of maintaining a trusting relationship.

An area which often causes trust to break down is in respect of communication. Working in collaboration with patients, service users, carers and other members of the interprofessional team inevitably requires good communication, consultation, and the disclosure and sharing of information. This aspect of care gives rise to two specific duties related to the value of trust and trustworthiness, those of confidentiality and truth-telling. Having to discuss personal and sometimes difficult, intimate and otherwise private information with relative strangers, calls for a degree of trust and confidence that the practitioners involved will respect the individual's privacy and confidentiality. Equally, patients and service users will expect practitioners to be truthful and honest when responding to questions and requests for information that informs their decision-making.

ACTIVITY 7.1

Think about a situation where you have placed your trust in another. This could be related to, for example, a personal friendship or someone who provides a particular service, e.g. a teacher, a plumber, or a healthcare practitioner.

- What was the nature of the trust you placed in them?
- What were the key components that you felt enabled you to place your trust in them? Why did you trust this person?
- Did you have any doubts about their trustworthiness? If so, why did you have doubts and what were they?

What you may have identified is a number of qualities of the individual, such as being reliable, being expert, having specific knowledge and skills or being competent, or something about your relationship with them, e.g. having confidence or being able to depend on them, even if they are relative strangers. All of these are connected with the notion of trust and in being trustworthy, i.e. that you deem them worthy of your trust. Another key aspect of trust that you could have identified is that you had confidence in trusting the person because they occupied a role that is recognised and certified by associations or professional bodies who define the competence or standard of their members, usually as a result of some specific training and education. Even something as simple as taking a taxi requires an element of trust; we can check that the driver is a registered cab driver which (hopefully) provides the assurance that he is qualified to drive. However, we have to trust that they will then drive safely, that their taxi is roadworthy and that the driver knows where he is going, and we may even trust that he will take the quickest (and therefore cheapest) route.

Trust exists in relationships where there are no absolute guarantees that a person has to act or behave in a certain way; if we could guarantee everyone's behaviour all of the time then the notion of trust would be redundant. For example, you expect that a car driver will slow down at a pedestrian crossing when the lights change to amber and will stop on red. In this case, the law expects this too and places a legal imperative on the driver. However, you also have to trust that the individual will observe the law and will stop at the red light; there is no absolute guarantee. Thus, trust is also 'dangerous' in that it involves *an element of risk*; the risk that either or both sides may let each other down or that you may lose what you have entrusted to another to protect or that people will act in ways that harm rather than benefit the trusting individual. For this reason, trust and relationships based in trust can also be misplaced and easily and irreparably damaged.

In trusting others we voluntarily place ourselves in a vulnerable position and we base our trust on the expectation that others will not take advantage of or exploit our vulnerability for their own self-interest and benefit, or for some misplaced understanding of our own good. This vulnerability may be accentuated in the therapeutic relationship, particularly if patients and service users feel apprehensive and intimidated by practitioners because of their apparent position of power and authority, resulting in an imbalance of control over decision-making and disempowerment. Self-respect can be shattered by a betrayal of trust (McLeod, 2006). You will find clear evidence of this if you read the Health Care Ombudsman's Report '*Care and compassion? Report of the Health Service Ombudsman on ten investigations into NHS care of older people.*' (Parliamentary and Health Service Ombudsman (PHSO), 2011).

Summary of conditions for trust

One's attitude is conducive to trust of another if there is:

- an acceptance of some level of risk or vulnerability (regarding whether they can be trusted to do what they are depended upon to do)
- an acceptance of the risk of being let down or betrayed (which is more than just being disappointed, e.g. you can rely on an alarm clock and if it breaks you are disappointed but not betrayed)
- an inclination to expect the best of the other person (at least in the areas in which you trust the person)
- optimism rather than pessimism or suspicion of the person to be trusted (but optimism and lack of suspicion can make one more open to harm)
- a belief or optimism that the person is competent (in certain respects)
- a belief or optimism that the person is committed to do what they are trusted to do
- a belief or optimism that, in general, the trusted person has a certain kind of motive for acting (controversial because unclear as to what motive we expect from people we trust)
- some expectation of shared moral values or norms and a moral disposition to be trustworthy; trustworthiness as a virtue.

Adapted from McLeod, 2006, pp.3–8

DIFFERENT TYPES OF TRUST

A distinction can be made between knowledge-based trust, trust in institutions and moralistic trust (Uslaner, 2001). We will also consider personal and professional trust.

Knowledge-based trust

A standard account of trust is that which depends on information and experience. On this account, we trust people because of our past experiences, knowledge and expectations of how they will behave or act, for example, in the knowledge that they have previously kept their promises, have been honest or have not betrayed our secrets. A single encounter of another is usually insufficient to establish your trust in the person; mutual trust develops through experience and is dependent on what we know about each other.

Trust in institutions

Trust in institutions has some similarities and some distinctive qualities. Institutions can include government structures and systems, healthcare organisations, hospitals, social services and professional bodies and groups. Putting faith in institutions may involve confidence rather than trust because institutions cannot reciprocate your trust in the same way as in individual relationships. However, we do make judgements about our trust in institutions according to our knowledge and experience. It is this trust in institutions that becomes threatened by reports of untrustworthy actions, malpractice and misconduct. In response we hear claims of increased governance, regulation, standards, transparency and accountability in attempts to regain or reinforce our trust in these institutions (O'Neill, 2002a). A culture of trust is equally important as trust between individuals. People thrive in an environment of trust (Gilson, 2006). Organisations that support a trusting culture are more profitable, have better teamwork and have happier staff.

Professional regulation is one significant measure used to define the responsibility and accountability of professional groups with a view to justifying public confidence and trust in the health and care professions.

ACTIVITY 7.2

- Find a Code of Practice relevant to your own practice setting.
- Read and examine the Code and identify how it endeavours to establish public trust and confidence. Are there clear statements about trust and being trustworthy or is this implied in other ways? Make notes outlining the key points identified.
- How do these statements relate to your own practice?

Trust is hard to define and apply to a whole group or institution; it may be easier from our knowledge and experience to say that we trust some nurses but not others, that we trust a doctor to treat one condition but not another. However, service users and patients rarely get to choose the practitioner who will provide their care; instead they place their trust in another because they are members of a profession or an institution. Being regulated and observant of a Code of Conduct goes a significant way to providing reassurance to the public. However, this is insufficient on its own to justify and prove the trustworthiness of individual practitioners. Although a professional is presumed to seek to fulfil policies, ethical codes, the law and their previous promises, unquestioning trust in members of a professional group can be misplaced; for example, as has been seen in the scandal uncovered at the Winterbourne View Review (DH, 2012b). Codes also only apply to a small proportion of the care workforce; a significant proportion of the health and social care team are not regulated by a professional body or bound by any specific code of conduct, and yet are likely to be involved in the intimate and personal aspects of an individual's care. There must be other reasons for placing trust in practitioners that goes beyond the membership of a profession.

Personal and professional trust

De Raeve (2002) debates the distinctions between personal and professional trust in the practitioner–patient relationship which has bearing on the discussion of the importance of trust placed in professions and non-professions. De Raeve (2002) claims that there is something distinct between those people with whom you have a personal relationship, e.g. a partner or close friend, those who are members of a trade or provide a service, and those who are 'professionals'. She makes the distinction between non-professional and professional work as being that between those occupations that require someone to be well skilled and know the facts and rules of the trade, and those professional occupations where judgement is also required and where rules can only operate as guidelines.

De Raeve (2002) takes this distinction further in establishing that it is the complexity and moral nature and implications of professional judgements that make the difference between the trust you might place in a tradesman in comparison to that invested in a health professional. For example, if a plumber is careless, he would be doing bad work on my house not on me and, although I may experience the consequences of his actions, his disregard for my interests is not the same as a doctor's or nurse's carelessness which may result in a direct harm to me which is morally reprehensible, regardless of the lack of intent (de Raeve, 2002, p.154). What is also important here is that the professional is held to account for their actions and takes responsibility for ensuring that I can rely on them; accountability is discussed in more detail in *Chapter 9*.

What also matters in the therapeutic relationship is the notion of moralistic trust or trustworthiness.

MORAL RESPONSIBILITY AND TRUSTWORTHINESS

We have already seen that trust in others may stem from our knowledge and experience and from their membership or belonging to institutions, such as professional groups or care sectors and services. To justify trust, practitioners must also take responsibility in their role, how their behaviour will influence and impact on individuals' lives and ensure that they can be relied upon. In placing their trust, service users and patients inevitably have to allow practitioners some discretion to fulfil their responsibilities; they have to rely, to some degree, on the expertise and knowledge of the practitioner. However, this does not give practitioners total freedom to do as they please and it is because of the risk associated with relying on others for care and support that trustworthiness is so important.

Moralistic trust

Moralistic trust is a moral commandment to treat people as if they were trustworthy (Uslaner, 2001). Thus, what is also fundamental to trustworthy behaviour is a strong sense and understanding of your moral values in relating to others, sensitivity and appreciation of their value positions and taking moral responsibility for your own judgements and actions in your everyday practice. Practitioners must be motivated to act in a trustworthy manner if they are to justify the trust placed in them (Smith, 2005, p.302).

ACTIVITY 7.3

- Make a list of the characteristics you believe are essential to being trustworthy.
- Ask three colleagues to list what they consider to be the key characteristics. Ideally ask people who hold different roles and responsibilities within the multidisciplinary team, e.g. a nurse, a social worker, a doctor, a counsellor, a therapist, a teacher.
- Compare and contrast your lists and discuss the similarities and differences with your colleagues.
- Try to think of reasons for the similarities and differences.

Trustworthiness is often referred to as a virtue (a quality of character that is morally good) and means being worthy of others' trust; that you will have a strong sense that morally right behaviour is important in your dealings with others. Being morally trustworthy also assumes that you will act according to appropriate moral norms and will have a good will or motive to your actions. Annette Baier (1986) connected this with a caring disposition.

Moral norms or values associated with being trustworthy include:
- demonstrating respect for others
- honesty
- integrity
- openness
- responsiveness
- caring for their wellbeing and having concern for their welfare
- being fair
- keeping promises and keeping confidences.

Trustworthiness also requires other interpersonal behaviours such as understanding others' individual experiences, communicating clearly and completely, and building partnerships (Thom and Campbell, 1997). People also expect that the trustworthy practitioner will respond in a moral way to their trusting behaviour and not betray their trust, i.e. that you will not take advantage of their vulnerability. Trusting a practitioner incorporates an expectation of a beneficial response, even though they could do harm (Smith, 2005, p.302).

Practitioners cannot simply assume that patients and service users will place trust in them solely because of the role they hold, be they nurse, doctor, social worker or care assistant. Demonstrating knowledge and competence alone is not enough for the development and maintenance of the trust which is so essential to the therapeutic relationship (Hupcey and Miller, 2006). Confidence in the organisation to provide reliable and competent practitioners provides a threshold of safe care from which trust can emerge but, although this is sufficient to be a reliable practitioner, trustworthiness must grow from this as you build the care relationship with the patient or service user. Given that different people's perceptions of trustworthiness will vary it is essential that care is individualised. Their trust will generally be well founded when the person they entrust is dependable, reliable and credible and willing to stand by their own moral standards, i.e. have moral integrity. Their degree of trust may be seen in their belief in your honesty, openness, reliability, sincerity, benevolence, kindness, compassion, selflessness and competence. This is a tall order for any practitioner. However, trust with patients and service users can take a long time to establish but can be destroyed in an instant through carelessness or a thoughtless act. It is therefore essential that you work hard to establish and maintain the trust of those in your care by practising with moral sensitivity, care, compassion and respect.

Two key areas of practice which are essential in establishing and maintaining trust in the care relationship are the principles related to confidentiality and truth-telling.

CONFIDENTIALITY AND TRUTH-TELLING

'Everyone using health and social care services in England is entitled to expect that information they entrust to care providers will be treated in strictest confidence. The promise of confidentiality has been a cornerstone of medical practice for centuries and the relationship of trust between a doctor and patient depends on it. The patient needs to be able to tell the truth about intimate matters, knowing that this information will not be improperly disclosed. This is equally important in social care.'

Fiona Caldicott and Kingsley Manning in the Foreword to the *Guide to Confidentiality in Health and Social Care*
(Health and Social Care Information Centre (HSCIC), 2013, p.6)

Introduction to the principle of confidentiality

The duty to maintain patient or service user confidentiality is fundamental to health and social care. It is enshrined in the law (Health and Social Care Act 2012) and further explained in the Health and Social Care Information Centre (HSCIC) *Guide to Confidentiality in Health and Social Care* (HSCIC, 2013) and in professional codes of practice and conduct. Practitioners have access to and are entrusted with wide-ranging information about their patients and service users and never has confidentiality been as important as in our increasingly technological information age.

Confidentiality has traditionally been associated with the one-to-one relationship between patients or service users and practitioners. However, with the introduction of single assessment processes and electronic records, greater clarity around confidentiality and the legitimate sharing of information is essential. The Health and Social Care Act (2012) made provision for the Health and Social Care Information Centre (HSCIC) to advise organisations on how to handle confidential information securely. Their *Guide to Confidentiality in Health and Social Care* (HSCIC, 2013) provides guidance for maintaining confidentiality and decision-making in difficult cases, through the application of five fundamental rules (see *Box 7.2*).

BOX — 7.2

Five rules for maintaining confidentiality

Rule 1

Confidential information about service users or patients should be treated confidentially and respectfully.

Rule 2

Members of a care team should share confidential information when it is needed for safe and effective care of an individual.

Rule 3

Information that is shared for the benefit of the community should be anonymised.

Rule 4

An individual's right to object to the sharing of confidential information about them should be respected.

Rule 5

Organisations should put policies, procedures and systems in place to ensure rules are followed.

Source: *Guide to Confidentiality in Health and Social Care* (HSCIC, 2013).

To help manage the risks associated with confidentiality or personal information, organisations are required by law to implement good governance practices which are based on a set of key principles: the 'Caldicott Principles'. The principles set out in the original Caldicott Report (DH, 1997) were revised as part of the Caldicott *Review of Information Governance in Health and Social Care* (Caldicott, 2013). This review of information sharing was undertaken to ensure that there is an appropriate balance between the protection of patient information and the use and sharing of information to improve patient care. When the original report was written in 1997, the health service was more paternalistic and less patient-centred. In 2013, Caldicott recognised that

'... citizens are a lot more concerned about what happens to their information; who has access to it, for what purposes is it used, and why isn't it shared more frequently when common sense tells them that it should be.'

(Caldicott, 2013, p.6)

The revised principles (see *Box 7.3*) provide a framework for making decisions about whether information should or should not be shared.

BOX — **7.3**

The Caldicott Principles

- Justify the purpose(s).
- Don't use personal confidential data unless it is absolutely necessary.
- Use the minimum necessary personal confidential data.
- Access to personal confidential data should be on a strict need-to-know basis.
- Everyone with access to personal confidential data should be aware of their responsibilities.
- Comply with the law.
- The duty to share information can be as important as the duty to protect patient confidentiality.

Source: Caldicott, 2013, pp.20–1.

Health and social care professionals should have the confidence to share information in the best interests of their patients within the framework set out by these principles. They should be supported by the policies of their employers, regulators and professional bodies.

In addition to the Rules and Principles identified in *Boxes 7.2* and *7.3*, it is recognised that opportunities for electronic health information exchange (eHIE) are changing rapidly. Many organisations share information through a third party called a Health Information Exchange. It is essential that patients understand how their information can be shared and have an opportunity to sign consent or to refuse consent for this to occur.

By law each organisation must appoint a named individual, a 'Caldicott Guardian'. This is a senior person within an organisation who is responsible for ensuring the governance and protection of confidentiality and who enables and guides appropriate information-sharing. The Caldicott Guardian plays a key role in ensuring that NHS, Councils with Social Services Responsibilities and partner organisations satisfy the highest practical standards for handling patient-identifiable information.

Defining confidentiality

ACTIVITY 7.4

Defining confidentiality

Think about the last time you told someone something 'in confidence'.

- Was there anything special or different about the information, and if so, in what ways?
- Why did you disclose this information and what did you expect of the other person/s with regard to this information?
- How did you convey your expectations with regard to how the other person would treat the information?
- Are you confident that the person did not disclose the information to anyone else? How would you feel if they had?

Use of the term confidentiality or telling someone something 'in confidence' generally implies an element of trust to keep secret that which is disclosed to a person or persons and usually pertains to private and personal information. If you think back to the discussion about trust, to trust another always involves an element of risk, so in sharing information in confidence you may well also attempt to protect yourself from risk by invoking a promise from the person you have confided in. How often have you said, 'I'll tell you this but you must promise not to tell anyone'? However, your belief in their trustworthiness is still important because you still have to trust that the person will also keep their promises.

Believing in the notion of confidentiality in itself therefore provides you with the confidence to share specific information that you would otherwise protect from the intrusion of others. In health and social care, individuals place significant trust in practitioners that the otherwise private and personal information that they share with you will be protected and they entrust this to you with the intent that it will be used for their benefit, for example to secure a diagnosis or to receive the appropriate care, support or advice.

Why is confidentiality important in health and social care?

Every day health and care workers are party to confidential information, usually given openly and willingly or acquired through the assessment process and care relationship. It would be near impossible to carry out accurate, effective and appropriate care without a certain amount of personal and private information about the patient or service user and they generally give it with the expectation that it will be used to their benefit. You are therefore in a privileged position to receive and be entrusted with this private information.

Consider the question, 'What information is subject to a duty of confidentiality?'

Confidential information is any information that is given to you in confidence and that is not freely available through normal social discourse. You have to be careful here because what you would disclose to others in normal conversation may not be the same standard as that set by the patient or service user. Certainly, any personal information related to their physical, mental and emotional health and wellbeing should be treated as confidential.

In English law, a duty of confidentiality will usually be recognised and information protected by equitable obligations of confidence if the following four criteria are satisfied (Herring, 2014, pp.224–6):
1. The information must be of a personal, private or intimate nature.
2. Information is given to another in circumstances which impose an obligation of confidence not to disclose the information, i.e. that the person receives information that they know or ought to know is to be regarded as confidential or private.
3. Where someone will suffer as a result of the release of confidential information about them or if it would be likely to cause a public harm, e.g. where a breach of confidence would result in a lack of public trust.
4. A breach of confidentiality would involve an unauthorised disclosure or use of the information.

The fact that individuals believe and trust that information passed to the practitioner will be kept a secret and hence is given with confidence is fundamental to the therapeutic care relationship. Service users and patients must believe that they can talk honestly and frankly without fear of exposure, otherwise they may withhold information important not only to their health, but possibly to the wellbeing of others. Jones (2003) found that patients clearly value confidentiality, see it as important to the medical consultation, and recognise that disclosure of information to others without their consent might deter patients from seeking treatment. However, the Information Governance Review (DH, 2013e) found that in the 12 months to the end of June 2012, 186 serious data breaches were notified to the Department of Health. Most involved the loss or theft of data, but almost one-third concerned unauthorised disclosures. This clearly indicates that practitioners are failing to meet the standards necessary for confidentiality.

ACTIVITY 7.5

Search for the HSCIC 'Guide to Confidentiality in Health and Social Care' (HSCIC, 2013) at www.digital.nhs.uk (accessed 19 January 2017; the Health and Social Care Information Centre is now hosted by NHS Digital)
- Read the rules identified and make some summary notes explaining each of these.
- Can you identify evidence of these rules being met in your care setting? Write down some examples.

What are the origins of a duty to respect confidences?

Confidentiality is one of the most deeply respected moral commitments in healthcare (Gillon, 1986). It is enshrined in many codes of practice, dating back to Hippocrates and the 'Hippocratic Oath' (originally sworn by doctors on entering the medical profession) which stated:

> 'Whatever, in connection with my professional practice, or not in connection with it, I see or hear, in the life of men, which ought not to be spoken of abroad, I will not divulge, as reckoning that all such should be kept secret.'

More recently, the modern version of the oath, the Declaration of Geneva (2006), extended this expectation of confidentiality to individuals even after their death, stating, 'I will respect the secrets which are confided in me, even after the patient has died.' Although much is written about medical confidentiality, by inference, and arising from their own professional codes of conduct and legal and moral principles, all other health and care practitioners are required to respect a duty of confidentiality.

Professional Codes of practice continue to place a significant duty on individual practitioners in health and social care to preserve confidentiality and not to reveal patient or service user information that is otherwise private and personal, although most codes suggest there may be some exceptions to this rule.

There are a number of reasons, aside from professional codes, why health and care workers have a duty to uphold confidentiality (Dimond, 2015, p.189):
- From the duty of care in negligence owed to those with whom you have a therapeutic relationship (this originates from the Common Law of Tort and negligence).
- From the implied duty under a contract of employment.
- From a duty to keep information passed on in confidence, confidential even when there is no pre-existing relationship or legally enforceable contract between parties i.e. a duty based on equity.
- From requirements by professional registration bodies as part of professional conduct, e.g. NMC.
- Duties created by statutes, especially the Data Protection Act 1998 and Article 8 of the European Convention on Human Rights 'Right to respect for private and family life' (Schedule 1 of the Human Rights Act 1998).

There is also a moral duty arising from the value of respect for persons and respect for privacy as a citizen and from the duty to promote their welfare through the development of a trusting relationship.

The moral value of maintaining confidentiality

The obligation to keep secrets arises from the value placed on respect for persons and their privacy, respect for their autonomy and the fact that harm may follow if the secret is revealed. We have already discussed the importance of people being able to have control over their own lives and make their own choices and this value extends to decisions about if, when and with whom their personal information should be shared. You have also seen that privacy is an essential component of maintaining dignity. Thus, if you are told a 'secret' it is usually knowledge that you have an obligation to conceal.

According to Garrett *et al.* (2001, pp.118–19) there are three types of obligatory secrets:
1. the natural secret
2. the promised secret
3. the professional secret.

The natural secret

The natural secret is so named because the information involved is by its very nature potentially harmful if revealed, e.g. private and intimate information. If the obligation to avoid harm is universal, i.e. owed by everyone, not just those in professional or contractual relationships, then even the lay person is obliged to keep such a secret; for example, that a friend has had a positive HIV test. However, there may still be exceptions where the risks of keeping such secrets outweigh those of disclosure, e.g. imagine a thief whom you caught red-handed saying, 'Ssh, don't tell the police, it's a secret!'

The promised secret

The promised secret is knowledge that we have promised to conceal. Generally, the promise exists because the information is also a natural secret. However, the particular harm associated with revealing a promised secret arises not only from the sensitivity of the information but also from the harmful effects of breaking promises. Deontologists may consider the duty to maintain confidences as a fundamental duty, regardless of a judgement of the consequences. They would ground this moral obligation in the duty of respect for persons, not using people as a means to an end, the right to autonomy and privacy and the duty to keep promises (fidelity). Deontologists also recognise duties associated with special relationships, such as those between a practitioner and patient.

Patients and service users may well assume that practitioners, simply through their relationship of providing care, have made an implied promise to keep their secrets, even when no express promise has been made. This is why it is particularly important to state that you cannot promise to always keep their information completely secret if there are circumstances where there may be some overriding duty to disclose and share the information, such as cases where it may place them at risk of significant harm. However, we generally depend on people in our social life to keep promises and most of us would be wary of the person we cannot trust to keep a promise, so exceptions have to be minimised.

The professional secret

The professional secret is knowledge that is obtained in a professional relationship that, if revealed, will harm not only the patient or service user but may also do serious harm to the profession and to the society that depends on that profession for important services. The duty to protect professional secrets is enshrined in the law or the code of practice but is also justified through the moral value of trust.

The importance of trust and the professional secret can be justified by contemplating the consequences of a loss of trust in the practitioner or professional group or service (consequentialist or utilitarian arguments). Consequentialist (utilitarian) arguments look to the harms and benefits resulting from maintaining confidentiality and the morally right action is that which serves the 'greater good'. If service users cannot trust you to keep their secrets they may feel betrayed and may be reluctant to disclose important information essential to their care, or it may prevent them seeking further support or treatment. This could result in care being inappropriate because it is based on inadequate or incomplete facts. Additionally, if a particular patient or service user reveals to others that their confidence has been breached, this may have a detrimental effect for the overall confidence in that service by other members of the public, ultimately putting the health and wellbeing of others potentially at risk.

The consequentialist would support the principle of respect for confidences as it would be desirable for the stability of society as a whole; without trust and respect, the fabric of society would be threatened. Also, people's health, welfare and general good and overall happiness will be better served if there is trust in health professionals. If people cannot rely on confidences being respected, they are less likely to seek medical help. For example, in the case of sexually transmitted disease and attendance at a genitourinary medicine clinic, the law prevents the disclosure of the patient's name in contact tracing, even to their general practitioner, without the patient's express consent. Therefore, it is in the interests of the individual and society that the patient can ask for advice in confidence. However, it is possible that the utilitarian could justify the need to tell or the breach of confidences based on the greater good of the majority or achieving the best available consequences or to prevent a greater harm. As you will see this is reflected in some aspects of law, e.g. statutes that either require or permit the breach of confidentiality in certain circumstances such as the control of notifiable diseases.

Thus there are very good legal, professional and moral reasons for valuing and respecting a duty of confidentiality. However, you may already be raising questions in your own mind as to whether or not you should always maintain confidentiality or whether there may sometimes be exceptions to this rule.

Is the duty of confidentiality an absolute duty?

In order to care in the most appropriate manner for patients and service users, and given that health and social care involves interprofessional, multidisciplinary and multi-agency approaches, it would be impossible for confidentiality to be an absolute principle. Nevertheless, any breaches of confidentiality should be exceptional and the duty of confidentiality should be a *prima facie* obligation (i.e. it must be maintained unless it conflicts on a particular occasion with an equal or stronger obligation).

ACTIVITY 7.6

Think about the incident of the thief whom you catch red-handed saying, 'Ssh, don't tell the police, it's a secret!' It would seem relatively uncontroversial to breach their confidence and report them to the police.

Now imagine that instead you come across this person while working in Accident and Emergency. They reveal to you that their injuries relate to a theft they have just committed but state, 'Please keep this a secret, promise you won't tell the police, I needed the money to pay for my child's school uniform.'

- Should you respect this patient's confidences in this case? Explain your answer.

- What exceptions are there to any duty of confidentiality?

As a practitioner you voluntarily undertake a general commitment to keep secrets and there is a contractual care relationship between the patient and practitioner that would justify maintaining the patient's confidences. Certainly, if you consider the value placed on respect for persons (regardless of their actions), then your first concerns would be the treatment and care required in relation to their injury. You may feel there is something intrinsically wrong with allowing illegal activity to go unheeded because of the harm they have caused to others, but there is no legal duty to report minor crime to the police and your duty to preserve the trust relationship should take priority. However, you should not purposely obstruct the police in their investigations, e.g. by giving false or misleading information and you can be required by a Court to give evidence or disclose relevant information through a court order.

Exceptions to the duty of confidentiality

It is accepted in law and in professional codes that confidentiality is a fundamental principle in health and care and there should be no use or disclosure of any patient or service user information other than for the care of the person to whom it relates. However, there are three broad exceptions to this standard that can be morally justified and which are recognised in the law and codes of practice (e.g. NMC, 2015; GMC, 2009), as well as specific legal requirements that impose obligations to breach confidentiality:

1. Consent – either implicitly for their own care or expressly for other purposes
2. Safeguarding
3. The public interest.

Consent

If patients or service users give their consent to the use or disclosure of information, then this gives you permission to breach their confidence. This is the least controversial of the exceptions, although it does assume the necessary conditions for consent have been satisfied, e.g. having capacity, being informed, and freedom in decision-making (the same conditions needed to making autonomous choices). Any disclosures should be kept to the minimum necessary and use anonymised or coded information if practicable to serve the purpose, e.g. audit of an aspect of care. The requirement of consent also means that you must honour informed refusal of consent to disclose. An individual's decision about whether information can be shared or not must be respected, except where this duty is outweighed by other more compelling obligations; such as safeguarding others or other legal requirements.

Safeguarding

The need to share information becomes an imperative in cases involving a threat to the safety of others. For example, this could involve the prevention of abuse to an elderly person or in cases of safeguarding children.

The HSCIC guidance on confidentiality provides the algorithm shown in *Figure 7.1* to help practitioners decide whether or not to disclose information.

The law of confidentiality applies to all adults as well as children where it can be demonstrated that they are fully informed, understand the situation and are judged competent to make a decision about the sharing or otherwise of confidential information relating to them. The term Gillick Competence is used in judgements of competence of children under the age of 16 years. This arose from the case of *Gillick* v. *West Norfolk Area Health Authority* [1986] AC 112 in response to the public policy requirement that some children should be able to access contraceptive treatment without necessitating the involvement of their parents. This case established that a child under the age of 16 years may be deemed competent to consent, providing they can demonstrate sufficient maturity and intellect to understand and appraise the nature and implications of the proposed treatment, including the risks and alternative courses of actions. These criteria would be applied to a child's ability to consent to the use or disclosure of information about them which gives you permission to breach their confidence.

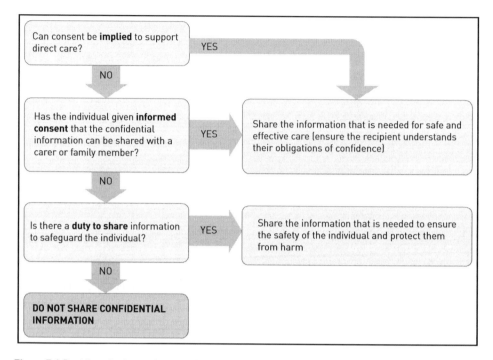

Figure 7.1 *Deciding whether to share confidential information for direct care. Reproduced from HSCIC, 2013, p.15, with permission from NHS Digital.*

If you work with children and young people you should also be aware of the importance of child protection law, particularly the Children Act 2004, and should be conversant with, and practise it at all times, in accordance with national and local policies and guidelines for safeguarding and protecting children and young people. The Mental Capacity Act 2005 generally applies to people who are aged 16 or older. However, Chapter 12 of the Mental Capacity Act 2005 Code of Practice (Department for Constitutional Affairs, 2007) explains how the Act affects children and young people, in particular those aged 16 and 17 years, and you would be strongly advised to read this if you work with children and young people in this age group. The Health and Social Care Act (2012) articulates requirements in respect of confidentiality.

Overruling the duty of confidentiality on the basis of acting in the best interests of the patient or service user is particularly challenging in cases where the capacity of an adult to determine for themselves what is in their best interests in a given instance is called into question. You need to think back here to the discussion of being autonomous, competence and respect for autonomy and the Mental Capacity Act (2005) in *Chapter 6*. Remember, you should always start from the position of assuming someone has the capacity to make a decision for themselves unless it can be established that they lack capacity.

Care must be taken when using judgements about mental capacity as a justification for breach of confidentiality. Think about this as you complete the activity in *Case study 7.1.*

CASE STUDY   7.1

You are the named care assistant for Tom, an 82-year-old gentleman who attends the Day Centre three times a week. He lives alone but has a son who calls in on him at home several times a week. Tom can be forgetful and sometimes gets confused about times of day and people's names, but he enjoys coming to the centre for the company of friends and joins in with all the activities. One day, he seems quieter than usual and you notice that he has some bruising on his forearms. When you sit down to talk to him, he tells you that a man has been coming to his house and has taken some money; you establish that this is probably his son. On further questioning, Tom says that his son can be a bit rough with him, but he implores you to keep this a secret because he loves his son and would not want him to get into any trouble, especially as he is so busy and helps him so much.

- What would you do in these circumstances?
- Would you be justified in breaching confidentiality in Tom's best interests?
- Discuss this case with colleagues and compare your responses.

You would obviously need more information in a case like this for you to make a truly informed decision as to whether or not you would be justified in breaching your duty of confidentiality. However, guidance on safeguarding would lead you to disclose this information to an appropriate authority to investigate further.

Public interest

There is also a moral, legal and professional exception to confidentiality where you can justify, in exceptional circumstances, that the rights to confidentiality are outweighed by the public interest, i.e. in order to serve a broader societal interest. Decisions to breach confidences in the public interest are complex and can be justified when the public interest in disclosure of information outweighs the public interest in protecting confidentiality. Because the public interest in maintaining the provision of confidential health and social care services is considerable (and is fundamental to trust in these services), breaches of confidentiality in the public interest should only be considered if there are weighty justifications to overrule the practitioner's prima facie duty of confidentiality, and these breaches should be kept to a minimum.

Justifications from the argument of the public interest include (Jackson, 2013, pp.384–99):
- preventing harm to others
- preventing or detecting crime
- teaching, research and audit
- statutory exceptions.

Preventing harm to others

If the risk of harm to others is used to justify disclosure, justification of a real risk of serious harm must be made. In cases where the individual concerned will not consent to disclosure, breaching confidentiality should only be considered if the threat posed is significant and imminent and disclosure can prevent or limit the expected harm (Jackson, 2013). The most frequently stated case in law that supports the rule of breach in the public interest is that of *W* v. *Edgell*, shown in *Box 7.4*.

BOX 7.4

W v. *Edgell* [1990] 1 ALL ER 835

The patient was a prisoner in a secure hospital following convictions for killing five people and wounding several others. He made an application to a mental health tribunal to be transferred to a regional unit. An independent psychiatrist, Dr Edgell, was asked by W's legal advisors to provide a confidential expert opinion that they hoped would show that W was no longer a danger to the public. However, Dr Edgell was of the opinion that in fact W was still dangerous. W's application was withdrawn. Dr Edgell, knowing that his opinion would not be included in the patient's notes, sent a copy to the medical director of the hospital and to the Home Office.

The patient brought an action (against Dr Edgell) for breach of confidence.

The Court of Appeal held that the breach was justified in the public interest, on grounds of protection of the public from dangerous criminal acts. However, the Court said the risk must be 'real, immediate and serious'.

Source: UK Clinical Ethics Network at ukcen.net/index.php/ethical_issues/confidentiality/legal_considerations (accessed 19 December 2016)

This case established that in order to justify disclosure in the public interest, you must prove:
- There is an imminent, real and serious risk of danger to the public (and can only justify disclosure as long as the threat persists).
- Disclosure must be to a person with a legitimate interest in receiving the information, e.g. 'the responsible authorities'.
- Disclosure should be confined to the disclosure of information that is strictly necessary (revealing some aspects of information in the public interests does not justify disclosure of all his/her details).

Therefore, you would be justified in breaching confidentiality in cases where the disclosure (Hendrick, 2004, p.124):
- would prevent serious risk of crime, e.g. murder, manslaughter, gun crime, child abuse

- would prevent threats to national security
- would prevent serious risk of harm, e.g. child abuse or neglect, spread of infectious disease, assault, serious fraud or theft
- is required by statute.

Statutory requirements

A number of statutes (law established by a legislative body, e.g. Acts of Parliament) create specific exceptions to the duty of confidentiality. Where a statutory requirement exists, patients' consent to disclosure is not necessary and they have no right to refuse. However, they should be made aware of the disclosure and that it is to a secure authority (BMA, 2009a, p.39). Some of the statutes are listed in *Box 7.5*.

BOX — **7.5**

When the law requires or permits disclosure of confidential information

Examples of disclosures required by statute include:

- Public Health (Control of Disease) Act 1984 and Public Health (Infectious Diseases) Regulations 1988 – a health professional must notify local authorities of the identity, sex and address of any person suspected of having a notifiable disease, including food poisoning.
- Abortion Regulations 1991 – a doctor carrying out a termination of pregnancy must notify the Chief Medical Officer, giving a reference number and the date of birth and postcode of the woman concerned.
- Reporting of Injuries, Diseases and Dangerous Occurrences Regulations 1985 – deaths, major injuries and accidents resulting in more than three days off work, certain diseases and dangerous occurrences must be reported.
- Road Traffic Act 1988 – health professionals must provide to the police, on request, any information which may identify a driver alleged to have committed a traffic offence.
- Terrorism Act 2000 – all citizens, including health professionals, must inform police as soon as possible of any information that may help to prevent an act of terrorism, or help in apprehending or prosecuting a terrorist.
- The Information Sharing Index (England) Regulations 2007 (ContactPoint) – health professionals must provide basic identifying information to the local authority for every child up to the age of 18.

Examples of disclosures permitted by statute include:

- The Data Protection Act 1998
- The Crime and Disorder Act 1998
- The Children Act 2004.

Source: BMA, 2009a, pp.39–40.

These permit disclosure to other organisations, such as the police, local authorities, social services, schools, Multi-Agency Protection Panels and government bodies. In these situations, health professionals may only disclose information when the patient has given consent or there is an overriding public interest. If health professionals have any doubts about whether the disclosure is a statutory obligation, they should ask the person or body applying for the information to specify under which legislation it is sought.

Breaching confidentiality is a serious issue and you should not be making this decision alone. If you are faced with a difficult decision you should approach the Caldicott Guardian for your organisation and area of practice who will advise on the individual case.

The HSCIC Guidance on Confidentiality (2013) identifies that three rules must be observed in any controlled breach of confidentiality:
1. The individual should be informed about how their information may be shared or used.
2. Steps should be taken to use the minimum level of confidential information necessary to support the purpose.
3. The law should be checked to ensure that there are no legal restrictions with regard to the sharing of information.

ACTIVITY 7.7

Use the following questions to guide your reflections on this section:
- Why do you think that confidentiality in health and social care is so important?
- How can you ensure it is protected?
- Why is confidentiality not an absolute duty?
- When must you obtain the patient or service user's permission to communicate with others about them?
- What would you do if a person revealed to you that they were HIV positive but refused to tell their partner or give you consent to share this information with any other practitioner?

If we value trust, then preserving the service user's right to confidentiality is one way of achieving this. However, there will be occasions when the arguments for disclosure will outweigh your duty to maintain confidentiality. What is important to minimising the loss of trust and helping to maintain the therapeutic relationship in these circumstances is that you reassure the patient or service user that they will still be cared for and that you are honest with them about why you must breach confidentiality.

Being honest and telling the truth is another fundamental component of being trustworthy.

THE VALUE OF HONESTY AND TRUTH-TELLING

Truth is an important value in our everyday lives; we do not want (or like) to be deceived and equally we find it difficult to deceive others. And yet, the value attributed to truth-telling is not as straightforward as it might at first appear. Even in our closest relationships, we choose what we will disclose and what will remain unsaid; maybe because we think our honesty would hurt, maybe to 'keep the peace', maybe because something would take too long to explain. Telling the truth relates closely with respect for the person as well as the value of trust in relationships. However, being honest is not necessarily easy, especially when we feel the truth may hurt those receiving it.

ACTIVITY   **7.8**

This exercise is intended to establish your attitudes towards the rights and wrongs of truth-telling with patients and service users. Think about the following questions in relation to your practice. Do you think all or only some are morally justified? Think of examples for each and about how you would justify your approach if called to account for your actions.

Are there circumstances:

- When you would *not* tell the truth?
- When you would tell a *lie*?
- When you would not tell the *whole* truth?
- When you would *force* the truth on a person, i.e. confront them with the truth for their own good?

Adapted from Downie and Calman, 1994, p.160.

Why should you tell patients and service users the truth?

The ordinary ethics of truthfulness according to Garrett *et al.* (2001, p.112) is encompassed in two duties: first, that you should not lie. Secondly, that you should communicate with those who have a right to the truth.

Yet, these seem far too simple to explain the complex problems met in real life where truth-telling and lying can be seen to be at two ends of a continuum, with evading the truth, deception and the notion of 'little white lies' falling in-between. The first statement seems to leave you free *not* to communicate (perhaps even to evade the question?) and the second raises the question, 'Who has the right to be told the truth?'. Neither statement says you must tell everyone everything you know or everything they want to know. However, we grow up believing (on the whole) that, 'honesty is the best policy'.

ACTIVITY (7.9)

Ask colleagues what they believe about being honest and telling the truth to service users/patients.

- Do they always tell the truth to service users/patients?
- If not, what exceptions do they identify? How do they justify not telling the truth?

Now find out the perceptions of friends and family regarding the importance of truth-telling in health and social care.

- Do they believe health and care practitioners always tell the truth to service users/patients? If not, why is this?
- Do they think practitioners should always tell the truth? Why?

Respect for people and their autonomy

Information giving is one of the necessary conditions to enable a person to be self-determining or autonomous and it is important that the information provided is honest and true (as far as we can know the truth at any particular point in time). If you restrict or withhold information that could otherwise inform the patient or service user's desires, choices and decisions, you are inevitably influencing (and possibly preventing) their opportunity to be autonomous. This reduces their ability to be in control of their lives and fails to show respect for persons. People need information not only to enable them to make autonomous choices but also to inform them about their situation regardless of whether there is a choice or decision to be made. The truth will help them to plan their care, seek support and attention when needed and to make life decisions that they would not make if they were unaware of their situation or condition.

The expectation of informed consent

It follows from the information condition of being autonomous that knowing the truth is also necessary for people to give informed consent. Giving consent in health and social care is a very real expression of the trust placed in the practitioner, as consent usually involves devolving some element of responsibility for that person's health and wellbeing to someone else.

Truth-telling may also be intrinsically good for the patient or service user

Telling people the truth may contribute generally to their health and wellbeing; for example, giving information prior to surgery has been shown to reduce anxiety and post-operative pain and improve recovery (see, for example, the seminal works of Boore (1978) and Hayward (1975)). Also, some people will simply find comfort in knowing that their symptoms can be attributed to a particular condition.

As one of the foundations of trust in the therapeutic relationship

If the person's expectations of being told the truth are met then this will contribute to their trust in those responsible for their care (which we have already seen to be fundamental to the therapeutic relationship). Consequently, they may also be more willing to cooperate with and seek treatment when required.

Is it ever right to withhold the truth?

> '... deception is the real enemy of trust.'
>
> (O'Neill, 2002c, p.3)

We generally believe that to deliberately deceive another, which includes withholding or distorting the truth or lying, is wrong. It is not just about getting the information wrong (which affects their ability to be autonomous) but is also about the motive and deliberate intention behind the deceit that is harmful to the person and their trust. If, in all honesty, you give the wrong directions to a stranger, they will find it annoying but not as much as if you had deliberately misled them for some personal pleasure or ends (O'Neill, 2002c, pp.3–4). Think about how you felt when someone has deliberately deceived you as a practical joke, or how you would feel if someone you secretly adored arranged to meet you for a date but without ever having the intention of turning up. In either case, you can imagine the humiliation, hurt, embarrassment, disbelief and anger that you might feel and it could well threaten your trust in the person that deceived you. As O'Neill (2002c, p.4) reminds us,

> 'It is because their falsehood is deliberate, and because it implies a deliberate intention to undermine, damage or distort others' plans and their capacities to act, that it damages trust and future relationships.'
>
> (O'Neill, 2002c, p.4).

From this you can see the close connections with the value of respect for persons and their autonomy because the deception and misinformation frustrates a person's ability to be autonomous. Being untruthful, evading the truth, deception and lying can also have serious consequences, both in the direct harms to the individual and through damaging their trust in therapeutic relationships or those with relatives and carers.

Thus, there are three different obligations related to truth-telling:
1. Not to lie
2. Not to deceive, and
3. To tell the truth.

To tell the truth appears, on the face of it, to be straightforward, although we could debate what the truth is in itself and certainly, in the current information age, the truth is becoming increasingly hard to know. It may be difficult to assess the 'truth' that should be told because of misleading or conflicting information. Sometimes too much information can be as disabling as too little when attempting to make informed choices and decisions. However, it is essential that you keep up to date with the available evidence related to your practice and learn skills in literature reviewing and discriminating between the validity and reliability of sources, particularly the plethora of information on the internet. This is important in supporting patients and service users who have difficulty in determining the authority and credibility of information. Of course, we may not always know the truth ourselves or be able to communicate the truth because of someone's incapacity to understand but this does not mean that you cannot still be truthful. To say, 'we don't know what is causing your symptoms' is being truthful (assuming this really is the case) even though it may not be what the person wants or needs to hear.

Truth-telling can be most challenging in caring for people with terminal or life-threatening illnesses. Practitioners may be concerned about the consequences of telling the truth and the ways in which this may cause harms such as anxiety and diminish feelings of hope for both the patient and their families (Clayton *et al.*, 2008; Pergert and Lützén, 2012). The 'truth' may include factual yet sensitive information about a new and serious diagnosis, treatment involving side-effects or a prognosis that moves from curative to palliative treatment (Pergert and Lützén, 2012). Conflict can arise between the wishes of the family to withhold information because they 'know the person best' and fear that their loved one will lose hope, while the practitioner believes it is their duty to be honest and to tell the truth. Withholding information about a person's diagnosis or prognosis can be seen as deceiving or misleading, even though a direct lie is not used.

Truth-telling obligations may become blurred in practice, particularly in cases where the truth seems potentially hurtful or when caring for people who lack mental capacity and the ability to distinguish between truths and falsehoods.

We cannot ignore the fact that to act in this way is an act of lying which is generally wrong, although the motive behind the lies and deception in each of these cases is (hopefully) one of avoiding harm and concern for the person's welfare (rather than one of self-interest, e.g. just making the job easier). There may also be some concomitant concerns for the welfare of others if the individual's behaviour is disturbing other patients, although careful consideration must be given to whether this justifies lying to one individual for the benefit of others.

Schermer (2007) argues that dementia slowly diminishes the capacities a person needs to distinguish between truths and falsehoods and with this, the ability to be lied to also disappears. However, outright lies to people with dementia should be avoided because they compromise the practitioner as well as threaten to undermine trust in care services. If we believe lying is fundamentally wrong (imagine what we would do if we thought

ACTIVITY 7.10

Truth-telling and the person with dementia

Read the following two examples taken from Schermer (2007, pp.14–15).

'Imagine a confused woman banging on the locked door of the ward, begging everyone in the neighbourhood to open the door so that she can go and collect the children from school. Telling her that her children are long grown up and are not waiting for her only worsens her agitation and confusion. So one of the nursing aides takes her arm and says, "Come on Mrs G, the children will not be out for another hour, let's go have a cup of tea first".'

(p.14)

'Another example is that of a widower who keeps asking about his wife, and who is inconsolable every time when he is told that she has passed away. Why hurt such a patient by confronting him with the painful truth time and again? Why not just distract attention by a small lie and tell the widower his wife is out shopping?'

(pp.14–15)

- What are your feelings about the suggested lying and deception in each of these hypothetical cases?
- Is lying justified? Explain your answers.

everyone might lie), the moral reasons to reject lying should apply equally for people with dementia. This may, however, depend on the capacities of the patient, such that lying may sometimes be justified on the count of caring for their wellbeing. Remember, to say something is 'just a little white lie' makes no difference; it is still a euphemism for lying (but trying to convey perhaps that the motive is not bad). As with many moral dilemmas, there are no easy, straightforward answers but, '… in general, methods that enhance the wellbeing of the patient without deception or lies should be favoured above options that use deceit, and methods of getting the truth across without hurting the patient should be favoured above blunt honesty.' (Schermer, 2007, p.13).

Any justification for deception or evading the truth becomes even harder to establish in cases where the patient or service user is fully competent and autonomous. Protecting the person from 'bad news', e.g. a diagnosis of chronic or terminal illness, even from a compassionate, well-intentioned concern for their welfare, would be paternalistic, i.e. acting in what you assumed to be their best interests even when they were capable of autonomous decision-making. We have discussed some of the problems associated with paternalism in *Chapters 5* and *6*.

Another argument sometimes mounted against truth-telling is that some patients and service users do not want to know the whole truth about their condition or prognosis because they would find it too burdensome. In cases where they are obviously autonomous and state their preference not to be told, it seems only right to allow them this choice and we should not force unwanted information on them (although lack of information to inform understanding and decisions may cause problems for informed consent). However, there is often a false assumption that patients do not or would not wish to be told the truth, even if it is unpleasant. Others may not ask but simply expect to be told more about their condition.

Friedrichsen *et al.* (2011) found that terminally ill cancer patients identified individual preferences from three different modes of truth:

- the absolute objective truth that they were dying;
- the partial truth about their condition including some facts but not all of the details; and
- the desired truth, originating in the patient's own beliefs about a healthy or better life.

The patients' coping strategies related to their preferred mode of truth. Some wanted to be faced with the absolute truth in order that they could take action and retain some sense of control. Others wished to face some parts of the truth in order to maintain hope, while others hovered between facing and avoiding the truth. Patients used different coping strategies, changing from one to another depending upon the circumstances. Thus truth-telling entailed more than merely providing information related to the person's forthcoming death. It was also concerned with how the doctors and other healthcare staff supported the patient and the need to fine-tune their communication of the 'truth' according to the individual patient's preferences.

One of the other difficulties is that one person's right to know or be told the truth may conflict with another person's right to confidentiality. For example, in cases of predictive genetic testing for Huntington's disease someone may choose to be tested because their grandparent has the disease but their own parent has chosen not to be tested. However, if the test proves the grandchild has the faulty gene, then this automatically means that their parent has it as well. Trying then to keep this result secret is likely to be difficult or even impossible for the person who has been tested.

ACTIVITY 7.11

Locate and read the following journal article:

Tuckett, A. (2004) Truth-telling in clinical practice and the arguments for and against: a review of the literature. *Nursing Ethics*, **11(5):** 500–513.

While reading, make notes that identify the arguments 'For' and 'Against' truth-telling presented by Tuckett's review of the literature.

- Do you agree with each of the arguments?
- Can you think of additional arguments? If so, add these to your list of 'For' and 'Against'.

Lies and deceptions may be used with the best intentions. However, it is important to first seek other ways of conveying the truth rather than resorting to using lies and deceit as the first line of action to avoid hurting the person in your care. To do this will require good interpersonal and communication skills and insight into the individual's understanding, capacity and circumstances and the range of possible alternatives available in any given situation. The risk associated with getting into the habit of being economical with the truth, deceiving or lying is that you will too easily resort to these practices when they are not justified.

CONCLUSION

Learning to be trustworthy may not be as straightforward as it sounds; it is more than being reliable and skilled to perform tasks or a role to some defined standard. Instead, it also requires you to develop a trustworthy disposition, with sensitivity to the values of the patient or service user and insight into the value they attribute to what they entrust to you, be it their personal and intimate information, their wellbeing, support or whatever this might be. It is essential, too, that you take responsibility for the effect you have on their perception of trust both in you and, as a consequence, in other practitioners and that you do not exploit the vulnerability and goodwill of the service user when they place their trust in you. Practising in ways that preserve and protect their privacy through your duty of confidentiality, being honest and not deceitful in your interpersonal interactions and respecting their autonomous choices through the consent process in care decisions are all ways in which you can foster trustworthiness and justify the trust service users place in you.

CHAPTER SUMMARY

Six key points to take away from Chapter 7:

- Building successful care relationships with service users and patients depends on trust.
- Trust and trustworthiness can be understood in a number of ways, including as an attitude towards other people or as a characteristic of individuals which can be described in moral terms and as a virtue.
- Maintaining confidentiality is one of the fundamental principles for trust in care practice. There are strong moral justifications, including respect for individual autonomy, promoting patient welfare and maintaining trust in the care relationship.
- Breaching confidentiality can be morally justified, or even required in some circumstances, i.e. in the best interests of the service user, in the public interest or when required by law. However, any breach should be exceptional and if a decision is made to breach patient confidentiality, the service user must be informed.

CHAPTER SUMMARY CONT'D

- Trust is generally promoted by honesty and truth-telling or undermined by deception; exceptions are rarely justified.
- One of the real expressions of a patient's or service user's trust is when they give informed consent for you to perform a procedure or do something on their behalf.

FURTHER READING

Department of Health (2013e) *Information: to share or not to share?* The Information Governance Review. London: HMSO.

Dinç, L. and Gastmans, C. (2012) Trust and trustworthiness in nursing: an argument based literature review. *Nursing Inquiry*, **19(3):** 223–237.

Health and Social Care Information Centre (HSCIC) (2013) *A Guide to Confidentiality in Health and Social Care.* London: HSCIC.

O'Neill, O. (2002) *A Question of Trust. The BBC Reith Lectures 2002.* Cambridge: Cambridge University Press. Available as transcripts at bbc.co.uk/radio4/reith2002/lectures.shtml (accessed 19 December 2016)

Sellman, D. (2006) The importance of being trustworthy. *Nursing Ethics,* **13(2):** 105–115.

PROTECTION FROM HARM AND PROMOTING INDEPENDENCE

In this chapter you will:

- consider your duty of care in protecting people from harm

- consider your responsibilities to provide safe and compassionate care and reflect on your obligation to raise concerns when individuals are put at risk

- reflect on the concept of risk

- apply the principles of risk assessment and risk management to the care context

- consider the value of independence versus protection

- apply the notion of planned risk-taking to the care context.

INTRODUCTION

Protection from harm and the promotion of best interests are concepts that are central to care work. Caring for another is a very responsible role. People in receipt of care are, as Sellman (2011, p.49) reminds us; 'more than ordinarily vulnerable' and they consequently need 'more than ordinary' support and protection. The public trusts practitioners to provide high quality, compassionate care for people who are in need and who may be at their most vulnerable; as a result of fear, illness, pain, frailty, lack of capacity or some other debilitating condition. In order for patients and service users to feel confident about receiving care they must be able to trust that the person caring for them will always act to maintain their safety, protect them from harm and as far as possible promote and support their best interests.

When safety and protection fail, it has a detrimental impact not only on those directly affected by the incident, but also more generally. The public lose confidence in services and in care practitioners specifically; trust of all practitioners is called into question.

Harm can take many forms. Harm can be characterised as hurt or damage and can be a result of an act (deliberate or accidental), or a result of failure to act, such as the harm that occurs in neglect. The protection and safeguarding of people in receipt of care services is everybody's responsibility. Protection from harm is articulated in laws designed to protect, in the values expressed in the NHS Constitution (DH, 2015a) and in various standards, such as the Care Quality Commission's (CQC) sixteen Essential Standards (CQC, 2010). Compliance with statutory and legal requirements is regulated through inspection from bodies such as Monitor, CQC (or Care Commission Scotland or the Healthcare Inspectorate Wales). These bodies have an increasingly important remit in regulating and monitoring care provision and in reassuring the public about standards of care they can expect to receive.

The regulators and inspectors are responsible for ensuring that organisations that provide care assume proper responsibility and accountability for providing good quality services. However, while these bodies fulfil an important role in inspecting care providers, the level of monitoring they can provide is insufficient to guarantee care safety, or to ensure that failures are addressed at the earliest opportunity. Safe care requires that every practitioner accepts the personal responsibility to ensure that they personally provide consistent, compassionate care and protection that meets best possible standards. It is also the practitioner's responsibility to be alert to the standards of care provided by others and to take positive action when these standards are called into question.

Trust in care services has been severely dented in recent years; a number of well-publicised care scandals and evidence of shocking levels of abuse and failures in care by practitioners have caused the public to question the compassion of those who provide care (Ombudsman Report (PHSO, 2011); *The State of Health Care and Adult Social Care in England* (CQC, 2013); South Gloucestershire Safeguarding Adults Board serious case review of Winterbourne View Hospital (Flynn, 2012); the Francis Inquiry Report (Francis, 2013)).

The appalling account of failures at Mid Staffordshire NHS Trust revealed in the Francis Inquiry in 2013 makes for harrowing reading. It raises the question: 'How could these failures and abuses have been tolerated for so long?' The outcome of the Francis Inquiry is a Report (Francis, 2013) with 192 recommendations for service improvement and it delivers a clear message to Government, care services and individual practitioners that failures of care, such as these, cannot be tolerated and action must be taken to prevent anything similar from happening again.

ACTIVITY **8.1**

- Read the Executive Summary of the Francis Report or the stories in the Ombudsman Report 2011 and reflect on how these situations could have been allowed to go on for so long.

Care and compassion? Report of the Health Service Ombudsman on ten investigations into NHS care of older people (PHSO, 2011). Available at:

gov.uk/government/uploads/system/uploads/attachment_data/file/247493/0778.pdf

Report of the Mid Staffordshire NHS Foundation Trust Public Inquiry Executive Summary (Francis, 2013). Available at:

gov.uk/government/uploads/system/uploads/attachment_data/file/279124/0947.pdf

Care, wherever it is delivered, must be safe, compassionate and meet the expectations of patients and their families. When care fails to meet these standards it is the responsibility of everyone, but specifically practitioners, to raise concerns and alert managers and other authorities at the earliest opportunity to ensure that lapses can be investigated and rectified quickly. The duty to 'protect from harm' is a very strong obligation in care practice and it is owed to all recipients of care by anyone who is contracted to provide care. People who use care services cannot always be cured or have all of the factors that make them vulnerable removed, but they should always be treated with compassion and respect and they should not, normally, be worse off as a result of experiencing care than they were before they received it. When a patient is harmed as a direct result of actions or neglect by practitioners this must be viewed in terms of abuse.

Different typologies of abuse have been identified by emerging research into this area.

- **Physical abuse** including hitting, slapping, pushing, kicking, misuse of medication, restraint, or inappropriate sanctions.
- **Sexual abuse** including rape and sexual assault or sexual acts to which the vulnerable adult has not consented, or could not consent or was pressured into consenting.
- **Psychological abuse** including emotional abuse, threats of harm or abandonment, deprivation of contact, humiliation, blaming, controlling, intimidation, coercion, harassment, verbal abuse, isolation or withdrawal from services or supportive networks.
- **Financial or material abuse** including theft, fraud, exploitation, pressure in connection with wills, property or inheritance or financial transactions, or the misuse or misappropriation of property, possessions or benefits.
- **Neglect and acts of omission** including ignoring medical or physical care needs, failure to provide access to appropriate health, social care or educational services, the withholding of the necessities of life, such as medication, adequate nutrition and heating.

- **Discriminatory abuse** including racist, sexist, that based on a person's disability, and other forms of harassment, slurs or similar treatment.

Guidance and the requirements for the protection and safeguarding of adults can be found in the Care Act 2014 (HMSO, 2014a).

The expectations of practitioners for protection of their patients from harm are clearly articulated in a number of statutory documents and it is important that you familiarise yourself with the standards and behaviours that are expected of you, in your context. See *Chapter 14* of *Care and Support Statutory Guidance* (DH, 2014f) and *Protection of Vulnerable Adults – principles of safeguarding* (DH, 2011).

While each individual document has a unique emphasis there are a number of key principles set out in the standards for protecting adults:
- **Empowerment** – the presumption that, where possible, any intervention or decision is undertaken in partnership with the person affected and is supported by informed consent.
- **Protection** – it is important to identify and plan support for those at greatest risk.
- **Prevention** – it is better to take action before harm occurs.
- **Proportionality** – proportionate and least intrusive response appropriate to the risk presented.
- **Partnership** – local solutions through services working with their communities. Communities have a part to play in preventing, detecting and reporting neglect and abuse.
- **Accountability** – accountability and transparency in delivering safeguarding.

In recognition of their position in society there are specific requirements for the protection of children and young people, set out in The Children Act (2004) and in the guidance document *Working Together to Safeguard Children* (Department of Education (DoE), 2013):

'… the action we take to promote the welfare of children and protect them from harm is everyone's responsibility. Everyone who comes into contact with children and families has a role to play.'

(DoE, 2013, p.8 para 8)

Safeguarding and promoting the welfare of children is defined for the purposes of this guidance as:
- protecting children from maltreatment
- preventing impairment of children's health or development
- ensuring that children grow up in circumstances consistent with the provision of safe and effective care
- taking action to enable all children to have the best outcomes.

The guidance on effective safeguarding arrangements in every local area should be underpinned by two key principles:

- Safeguarding is everyone's responsibility: for services to be effective each professional and organisation should play their full part.
- A child-centred approach: for services to be effective they should be based on a clear understanding of the needs and views of children.

Protection from harm is clearly implicit within a 'duty of care' and it therefore falls within the remit of anyone undertaking a caring role. As discussed in earlier chapters, each practitioner must promote and respect the dignity, confidentiality and individuality of each person in their care and must act towards them with compassion, kindness and care. Each practitioner is also legally bound to raise any concerns, through appropriate channels as soon as they become aware that individuals are not receiving the care of a standard to which they are entitled. Each organisation will have a policy for raising concerns, or whistleblowing, and it is important that each practitioner familiarises themselves with their local policy.

ACTIVITY 8.2

Locate your policy for whistleblowing or raising concerns. Make sure you are familiar with your organisational policy and procedure for raising concerns.

Harm, however, does not just occur when someone's vulnerability is exploited or ignored. Harm also occurs when a practitioner fails to undertake necessary actions. Harm due to failure to act is easily understood when a practitioner fails to attempt to resuscitate someone who should have been resuscitated, or when there is a failure to administer prescribed life-saving medication. What is less clearly understood is the impact of the smaller, and some might say, less significant acts or failures which impact on the care experience.

Findings from research in the 1980s and 1990s into care and failures to provide compassionate care are as relevant today as they were then (see *Table 8.1*). It is important for practitioners to reflect on the quality of the care they provide and to think about how minor failures and strategies designed 'to get the work done' are experienced by those being cared for.

ACTIVITY 8.3

Read the summary of research findings about standards of practice in *Table 8.1* and think about your own practice. Be honest with yourself – have you ever engaged in any of the behaviours listed? If so, what do you think causes you to act in this way and what strategies could you put in place to prevent this in the future?

Table 8.1 *Summary of research findings on standards of practice*

Not so good care	Bad care
• Routine care	• Not respectful/patient not listened to
• Patients have to ask for help	• Careless
• Distant relationship/little rapport	• Failure to perform basic care activities
• Limited information	• Not treated as 'whole' human
• Lack of kindness or concern	• Inattentive
• Staff inaccessible/unavailable	• Have to wait
• Person does not feel cared about	• Forgotten/broken promises
	• Misjudgement
	• Inflexible routines
	• Abuse/neglect
Non-caring	**Uncaring/incompetent**
• Hurried/too efficient	• Depersonalise patients
• Not thoughtful	• Increase patients'
• Just doing a job	vulnerability/dependence
• Rough	• Neglect patients
• Belittle patients	• Detached
• Not responding	• Non-communicative
• Not paying attention	• Negative communication
• Treat patients as objects	• Indifferent
• See patients as problems	• Fail to meet care responsibilities

You should note that to experience poor care, it is not necessary for a person to feel that they are being maltreated or abused. If the practitioner is rushed and does not take time to provide a kind and individual experience, the care experience will be a negative one. Lack of time is often cited as an excuse for poor care. This may be a reason but it is not an adequate excuse. Lack of time is an individual practitioner or organisational issue, not the patient's issue. The patient needs to be protected from feeling harassed and a burden because the practitioner is busy.

Promoting independence is an important component of the duty of care; harm can result from over-protection and failure to promote independence. Of course, in order to promote independence, it is necessary to take risks and when you take risks there is always the possibility that it will result in harm. This is the tension that practitioners have to juggle. Where are the boundaries between protection and managed risk? There are no easy answers and each case will need to be assessed on its own merits.

We live in an increasingly risk-averse society; that is, one in which the belief is held that all risks should be anticipated and eliminated. The problem with this approach is that it can support excessive caution and can give legitimacy to unlikely risks. This in turn results in restrictive and over-protective practice. The care worker must constantly balance the competing demands of care so that it is neither over-protective nor too risky, but is instead care that promotes independence and self-governance for the patient.

The promotion of best interests

Protection from harm has been a long-standing responsibility of practitioners who provide care. In the past the articulation of the protection from harm principle was frequently interpreted as 'the promotion of best interests'. That is, it was the responsibility of the practitioner to determine best interests on behalf of the patient; usually based upon what they determined would be best for the patients' physical recovery or rehabilitation. This focus on the physical, to the detriment of other values and concerns, arose out of the primacy of the 'medical model of care'. This model implies that practitioners – doctors in particular – know what is in the best interests of those in their care, and that they are best placed to action those best interests, which is interpreted to mean that which fosters longevity. Inevitably this approach led to a paternalistic or parental approach to care practice, in which the practitioner had licence to tell the client what to do, and to expect the client to comply with those directions. Increasingly, this approach to care practice has come to be seen as problematic. This approach has a tendency to identify people by their illness or disability and care decisions are focused almost exclusively on that aspect of the person, rather than care that is designed to meet the many and varied needs and preferences of individuals; some of which may have nothing to do with the service user's physical health but which support people's right to determine preferences in their own life. If care is focused exclusively around illness rather than on individuals, it is difficult to accommodate individual differences and preferences. It is our individuality and the personal choices about how we live our lives that bring value to our life.

While the 'best interests' approach to care has fallen out of favour in recent times, it is important to note that it can have a place in care practice as long as it is selected with caution and with an appropriate rationale. There are times when an individual is too weak, or too compromised, to make decisions about their care for themselves, and they may ask you to act in their best interests. There are also times when, where safety is concerned, best interests, in the form of paternalism, is the fundamental reason for undertaking an action that protects someone from danger. The important thing to remember when applying a 'best interests' approach, that favours a paternalistic stance, is that it should be used only with a robust justification and when alternative approaches are unavailable. Practitioners should be constantly alert to supporting service users' rights to take back control of the decision-making in care at any point, or as soon as they are able to do so.

Increasingly our understanding of the role that practitioners play in providing care is being challenged by fundamental philosophical and social changes that require practitioners to engage with patients and service users as unique individuals for whom one rule of care cannot be applied. This social change is clearly reflected in government policy, which promotes the idea of independence and choice in care. The NHS Constitution (DH, 2015a) makes the commitment that patients, carers and the public will play a central role in determining services, and working in partnership with care providers who will be accountable to the public more overtly:

- **Principle 4:** The NHS aspires to put patients at the heart of everything it does.
- **Principle 7:** The NHS is accountable to the public, communities and patients that it serves (DH, 2015a, pp.3–4).

The following section will explore the concepts of protection from harm and the promotion of independence within the context of an increasingly risk-aware and risk-averse society. In addition, it will seek to provide practical examples of how care workers can both protect patients from harm and promote independence.

WHAT IS RISK AND DO WE NEED TO BE PROTECTED FROM IT?

Risks are part of our everyday experience; it is hard to imagine any activity that does not involve an element of risk. We learn from a very early age about risk assessment and risk-taking. Initially, this might be simplistic and might not be done at a conscious level. For example, children constantly test boundaries with their parents and risk censure in order to see what they can get away with. In this way they learn how to make risk-based judgements. As adolescents and adults we continue to learn from our experiences and improve our decision-making ability. We develop a bank of information that we can draw upon to help us make decisions when we face the same, similar or new situations in the future. When we are exposed to opportunities and experiences that we have never encountered before we make some assessment of the activity and decide whether or not this is a risk that we want to take. Without engaging in risk-taking it is impossible to become independent. Therefore, the notions of risk-taking and independence are inextricably linked.

Defining risk

Although risk-taking behaviours are, and always have been, part of our everyday lives, and although risk is essential for growth and development, risk and risk management have become a preoccupation and, some would say, the dominating feature of life in the 21st century (Denney, 2005) and yet there is no real consensus on the definition of risk.

Risk, with its early Arabic origin, *risq*, was a term used to denote outcomes that can be either positive or negative (Alaszewski *et al.*, 1998). However, by the time risk became part of the English language in the 15th century it had taken on a purely negative connotation and was primarily linked to the idea of hazards.

The fact that these hazards were seen to be beyond human control, i.e. acts of God or fate, meant that although they needed to be noted, primarily so that insurance in losses to shipping cargoes could be determined, no other preventative action was needed.

Even though risk was understood as a negative thing it was tolerated as a natural part of life. In recent years, risk has come to be seen as something that should be predicted, prevented, avoided or managed.

Why are we so risk-conscious?

There are a number of theories about why our attitude to risk has changed so radically in recent years:

- that we are exposed to more risks now than in the past, and that these risks are of a more devastating nature (Beck, 1992)
- that the knowledge revolution now means that we have the knowledge to understand and prevent risks that were not possible in previous times
- the increasingly secular society means that we can no longer blame God for what happens to us, but must be reliant on our own resources
- the individualisation of western societies means that we must be responsible for our own actions and behaviours.

Whatever the reason, we are constantly bombarded by warnings of the need to be aware of risks and to act responsibly. The daily reminders of risks regarding global warming, terrorism, the dangers of speeding, of sunbathing, of eating too much, getting fat and of taking too little exercise, of the vulnerability of children, etc. are endless and all give us the impression that life is dangerous, that risks are bad and that we must take precautions and avoid them; that wherever possible we should be adopting the 'better safe than sorry' principle (Furedi, 1997).

While much of this is good advice and can to some extent explain why we enjoy healthier, longer lives than ever before, it would be a mistake to believe that risk can, or should, be eliminated. What has been lost in the modern understanding of risk is the idea of positive outcomes.

ACTIVITY **8.4**

Remember a time when you took a risk in order to do something that you really wanted to do. Perhaps it was riding on a particularly high roller coaster, or driving on your own for the first time, or skiing down a steep mountain or risking doing a performance in front of an audience, or when you attempted something you never thought you could do. Whatever the activity you have in mind, remember the thrill and excitement of undertaking that activity, remember the sense of achievement and self-belief when that activity went well.

Risk-taking can be thrilling, and taking risks frequently does have a positive outcome. Without risk life would be boring; humans would cease to grow and to develop. If you apply this idea to the context of health, many of the positive outcomes in terms of treatments and advances in medicine have only occurred because someone took a risk. The sense of achievement is present whether it is a small risk taken by a patient or a much bigger risk to test a breakthrough in medicine.

Risk in health and social care

Why is all this relevant to the care practitioner? In protecting those in our care from harm, it is all too easy to focus on the negative side of risk. This inevitably causes us to practise in a defensive manner and to err on the side of caution. For example, we may seek to restrict the free movement of someone who has been known to fall but, while this may keep them safe, it fails to acknowledge their right to independence; over-protection means that their mobility may deteriorate still further and their confidence and sense of self-esteem may be seriously affected. In this case the practitioner can consider a number of questions relating to the key question: 'In what ways can I assist this person to more safely maintain their independent mobility?' After all, it might be necessary to acknowledge that absolute safety is unrealistic and that suitable preventative activities to reduce risk are the only really appropriate methods of addressing the issue. Therefore, the questions to ask might be:

- Does the individual have appropriately supportive shoes?
- Are there any walking aids that would offer support but enable the person to retain their independence?
- Is the environment safe?
- Are there any unnecessary obstacles that hinder the individual's mobility?
- Could the individual be offered an assessment with a physiotherapist to learn some strategies for greater stability?

These are just some of the strategies that can be explored. It may be easier to protect an individual, but good care emerges from looking at the problem and trying to find solutions not to eliminate the risk, but to manage the risk more effectively.

At times, risk assessment is undertaken at an organisational level and results in the development of a policy in relation to a specific issue.

The fear of blame

The risk focus in our society today is largely motivated by fear of blame. Part of our risk assessment will entail an analysis such as the following: 'If I let this activity go ahead what will happen if I have made a poor judgement and something goes wrong?' These worries may be partly on behalf of the person in our care, but equally may be worries about ourselves. If I make the wrong decision will I be blamed? What will happen to me? The increasing threat of being sued has resulted in an ever-increasing number of policies that effectively reduce the opportunities for individual practitioners to take independent decisions. Some of this is beyond our control and is a reflection of the society we live in. However, it is a useful exercise when we seek to protect, particularly in respect of restricting others' activities and freedom, to think about the following questions:

- Who am I protecting and why?
- Is the level of restriction appropriate?
- Do the benefits outweigh the disadvantages?
- Are there any other ways to manage the issue?

The growth of protective policy is part of the wider governance agenda that seeks to improve standards and protect those in our care through standardisation of the behaviours of practitioners. Governance is one response of the health and care sector to a series of public scandals in the health and social care arenas. Governance is also driven by an increasingly knowledgeable, but cynical, public whose expectations are significantly higher than they were twenty years ago, and who will seek compensation for errors of judgement. Governance is therefore an attempt to reassure the public of the safety and efficacy of the services that are provided. Risk assessment and risk management are key elements of that process. A central theme of governance is to develop a culture in which organisations and individuals are able to look at risk proactively. To ensure that good policies and procedures are in place to protect individuals and prevent accidents from happening, to analyse accidents, to learn from mistakes and then to further improve policies and procedures. Ideally it should promote a culture of openness that encourages individuals to admit their mistakes and errors in order that prevention in the future can be implemented. This can only be achieved if an organisation is able to convey the message that the investigation of mistakes is not to apportion blame, but is rather to learn from mistakes.

RISK ASSESSMENT

Risk assessment is now a daily activity within the care sector. Risk assessment requires a practitioner to think through the consequences of their decision-making and their actions, and make judgements on the basis of this activity. When engaging in risk assessment, practitioners are encouraged to assess the nature of the risk posed, as different types of risks need to be treated in different ways.

Predictable and preventable risks

Risks that are predictable, likely to be frequent and/or avoidable are issues that require us to put preventative strategies in place. These strategies may be seen as 'good housekeeping'. These risks should be anticipated and changes in practice should be implemented to prevent or reduce their incidence. An example of dealing with this type of risk is measures to try to protect service users from acquired infections. Procedures for hand washing and the widespread introduction of alcohol hand rubs are measures that have been introduced to reduce a known and frequent risk.

Risk assessment leading to 'policy implementation' is also used as a means to protect individuals from infrequent but potentially significant harm, for example, fire safety procedures. All organisations have well-established policies and procedures that would come into play in the unfortunate event of a fire. Staff are trained in the implementation of the policy on a regular basis, even though many will never have to put it into practice in reality. However, the training and knowing what to do if a fire happened could save lives and it is, therefore, an investment worth making.

Assessing individual risk

Risk assessment can also be applied to individual situations – assessing individual risk. This may be a one-off or a regular activity that relates to a specific person or group of service users. Assessing individual risks should be part of the day-to-day planning and care of people. However, the mindset that the practitioner adopts, in relation to risk assessment, will determine what decisions will come out of the assessment. If the practitioner sees danger in situations that are not completely within their control, then they are likely to risk-assess in a defensive and restrictive manner, and may decide not to engage in an activity at all. This is certainly what has happened in relation to the provision of school trips: because of a few widely-publicised problems that have occurred, teachers are increasingly reluctant to arrange trips, believing that abstaining from them is the most appropriate preventative strategy.

However, if the practitioner approaches risk assessment from a positive perspective, seeing risk as an essential part of life that must be engaged with and managed, then the risk assessment and the strategies that ensue from that will mean that the activity is less likely to be prevented and may be conducted in a safer manner than if no risk assessment had been made.

ACTIVITY 8.5

Imagine you are working in a rehabilitation or care home environment.
- Plan a trip/visit out with someone in your care. What risks do you think you are likely to expose the client to? Are there risks to you? Are there risks to others?
- Can any of the risks be reduced?

Doing a risk assessment is very likely to throw up all manner of potential risks and might discourage the care worker from engaging in the activity. However, it is very important to be able to distinguish between real risks and possible but unlikely risks (virtual risks). Remember what it feels like to take risks and to do the things that you really want to do. If you enjoy the sensation of risk-taking then so too will the person in your care. Taking reasonable and well-thought-through risks with service users is likely to give you, and them, a positive sense of achievement, but will also provide them with an opportunity to experience those things that bring quality to life. Living a life that is completely predictable and one hundred per cent protected is a very depressing thought. If viewed as a positive opportunity for safe practice, risk-taking may enhance the care of individuals and consequently enhance their life.

ACTIVITY 8.6

From your own experience list examples of:

- Risks that are managed through 'good housekeeping'
- Policies that exist to combat infrequent, but significant, potential risk
- Risk assessment of individual client issues.

The fact that a risk is likely or that a risk could have significant impact, does not necessarily mean that we should not engage in the risk. However, it does of course mean that additional care needs to be taken and the activity needs to be planned in order that the risk is minimised to an acceptable level and individuals and organisations are reasonably protected.

PREDICTING RISK

It should be noted that many risks are very difficult to predict accurately (Gale *et al.*, 2003; Titterton, 2005). It is commonly assumed that risk can be predicted through the application of objective assessment, reasoning about evidence and the prediction of likelihood and probability. However, risk assessment is not simply a matter of calculating the likelihood of an action happening and assessing the likelihood and magnitude of the potential harm that could result from taking that risk.

ACTIVITY 8.7

- Think about the risks of the following in your own life and try to predict the probability of them actually happening. For example, winning the lottery is well known to be a chance of somewhere in the region of 1:14 million.
  - Being burgled
  - Developing dementia
  - Being involved in an aeroplane crash.
- Check your answers with those below. How accurately did you predict the risk?
- Ask five other people the same questions. Discuss the similarities and differences in your answers. Can you identify any reasons for differences?

Answers to risks:

Risk of burglary 1:50 (higher in some areas than others)

Risk of developing dementia 1:14 in those over age 65, rising to 1:6 in those over 80

Risk of an aeroplane crash 1:4.8 million

Some risks have been the subject of significant research and we can predict fairly accurately the incidence or possibility of an occurrence happening. For example, our knowledge of epidemiology will fairly accurately be able to identify the statistical risk of contracting a disease, whereas there is insufficient evidence to predict the likelihood of me falling and breaking my leg. However, the incidence of a disease in the population does not help me to understand what that risk really means to me. My understanding of the risk will depend on how well I understand numbers and ratios, statistics and probability. Even if I do understand the figures, my interpretation of them will depend on a variety of factors and will determine whether I see the risk as a deterrent or an encouragement. For example, I might be tempted to play the lottery, because a 1:14 million chance is better than a 1:0 chance if I do not play. However, if the risk of 1:14 million applied to the risk of me contracting a disease, I would interpret that as being negligible and would not think that I needed to bother about it. However, someone else might see that as a real risk and take precautionary action. These differences in understanding and interpreting risks are known as risk perception.

Risk perception

The increasing concentration on risk in society has caused social scientists to explore the way in which individuals assess risk and what influences differences in people's perceptions of risk.

Risk perception involves people's beliefs, attitudes, judgements, experiences, and feelings, as well as the wider social or cultural values and dispositions that people adopt, towards hazards and their benefits (Pidgeon *et al.*, 1992, p.89).

Factors that affect our risk assessment and subsequent behaviours include:
- Our personality type – some people are naturally more cautious than others.
- Joffe (2003) asserts that individuals have an unrealistically optimistic belief that their future holds few adverse events.
- Women are generally less keen to take risks than men (Karakowsky and Elangovan, 2001).
- If an individual has positive feelings about a particular thing, because of past experience, personal values or unrealistic beliefs, then their risk assessment will be significantly different from someone who has negative feelings about a particular issue.
- Primacy – if there has been a great deal of publicity about a particular topic, or this is associated with very striking, disturbing or unpleasant effects, this will normally inflate your assessment of the frequency of the risk occurring (think, for example, about your own risk assessment of catching bird flu). People tend to overemphasise death from infrequent causes such as bird flu or BSE and

underestimate their risk of death from frequent causes such as cancer or heart disease (Pidgeon *et al.*, 1992).

- Fear of blame is likely to cause an individual to overemphasise the risk involved in an action.
- Some persons are perceived to be at more risk than others such as, for example, children or older people, while others are perceived to be more of a risk than others such as, for example, those with mental health problems or those who take drugs (Kemshall and Pritchard, 1996).
- The views of others – our notion of risk is impacted on by dominant beliefs and values in our culture and by those in our social groups and networks who will influence how we understand and relate to risk. This is known as the social construction of risk.

Differences in risk perception and individual responses to risk mean that any objective measurement of risk is only partially useful. It means that I am unlikely to make an accurate assessment of your preparedness to take a risk if I do not spend time finding out how you feel about an issue or how you interpret risk factors. The same applies to clients in our care. All too often, care workers make assumptions about what is best for individuals in their care without ever really discussing with them whether this is so. Risk cannot and should not be eliminated. What is relevant is ascertaining which risks are appropriate to take and in what way.

ASSESSING RISK IN PRACTICE

There are lots of different tools and pro formas for assessing risk in practice. Risk assessment has become an important element of care practice. Assessment tools such as the Waterlow Pressure Score Assessment (2005), the National Early Warning Score (NEWS) to identify deteriorating patients, nutrition assessment or Falls Risk assessment may be familiar. Risk assessment tools ask the practitioner to use a validated measure and apply data gained through observation and measurement to make an objective assessment about the level of risk to which a person may be exposed. These tools, and others like them, help the practitioner to determine the likely level of risk and to put in place interventions that avert or more effectively manage the risk.

You may also be required to answer questions similar to these when assessing whether or not to support an activity or intervention that carries some risk:

- Is the risk a real risk?
- Why is the risk activity proposed?
- Is there a good justification for the risk activity?
- What advantages are there of engaging in this activity?
- What could go wrong and for whom?

- How could this happen?
- What could the effect be?
- How severe will this effect be?
- How likely is it that this will happen?

Involving the service user in risk assessment

Questions such as these will help to build up a picture of the costs and benefits of a particular activity. Ironically, risk assessment is seen as the domain and responsibility of the care worker. There is scant evidence in risk assessment literature of the active involvement, and account taken, of the views of the service user themselves. However, you should, wherever possible, ask service users:

- What is the individual's / family's view of the risk?
- How important to the individual is taking this risk?
- How willing is the individual to risk a negative outcome?

Risk assessment requires practitioners to make judgements about another's capabilities, about the potential gains for the individual concerned, the potential disadvantages or harms of the risk, the values placed on the outcomes and the consequences of not going ahead with the risk (Titterton, 2005), but this cannot be done in isolation from the service user. Having made an assessment, the outcome of the assessment should be discussed with the service user and other members of the team to determine if the risk should be engaged in and/or if a risk plan can be put in place to take reasonable precautions to limit any negative outcome.

Using risk assessment tools

ACTIVITY 8.8

Using the structured risk assessment tool in *Figure 8.1*, recalculate the risk assessment for taking a client out on a visit that you did in *Activity 8.5*. Has your risk assessment changed?

Risk assessment tools do not necessarily provide the right answer. They are there to provide you with prompts to help to ensure that important issues for consideration have not been forgotten. Their use provides evidence of the assessment process that you have undertaken and demonstrates that you took the risks seriously. It should be remembered that accidents, mishaps and risks cannot be prevented. What is relevant is that we approach activities responsibly and with risks in mind so that we may be able to minimise the risks to which individuals are exposed.

Location/Service user(s) name(s) as appropriate:

Date:

Assessor:

1. Brief description of activity/issue and rationale for why the risk activity is proposed:

2. What are the benefits of engaging in this activity and for whom?

3. What is the significance of each of the benefits? Rate them on a 1–5 score with 5 = very important and 1 = not at all important. (Discuss the results with other relevant staff and the client/family.)

Benefit	Significance
	1 2 3 4 5
	1 2 3 4 5
	1 2 3 4 5
	1 2 3 4 5

4. Who benefits, how do they benefit and how likely is the benefit?

Who might benefit?	How might they benefit?	How likely is the benefit? (1 = not at all likely to 5 = very likely)			
		1	2	3	4	5
		1	2	3	4	5
		1	2	3	4	5
		1	2	3	4	5
		1	2	3	4	5

Total benefits score =

5. What risks/hazards could result from the activity? (Consider risks to the service user, the practitioner and the organisation.)

6. What is the significance of each of the risks/hazards? Rank them, with 1 being not very significant and 5 being very significant.

Risk	Significance				
	1	2	3	4	5
	1	2	3	4	5
	1	2	3	4	5
	1	2	3	4	5

7. Who might be harmed, how might they be harmed and how likely are they to be harmed?

Who might be harmed?	How might they be harmed?	How likely is the harm? 1 = highly unlikely 3 = can be reasonably foreseen 5 = highly likely				
		1	2	3	4	5
		1	2	3	4	5
		1	2	3	4	5
		1	2	3	4	5

Total risk score =

8. Compare the risks and benefits overall. Does either of the scores suggest that benefits outweigh risks or vice versa?

> **9. What (if any) strategies could be put in place to make the activity safer?**

> **10. If these strategies are put in place, does this change the risk assessment score?**

> **11. What is the overall score, having taken account of the effects of strategies that can be implemented to minimise the risks?**
>
> Benefits =   Risks =

> **12. Decision on action to be taken and reason for decision:**

Signed:

Practitioner _____   **Service user** _____
                                                 (or approved representative)

Figure 8.1 *Risk assessment tool for managed positive risk-taking.*

RISK MANAGEMENT AND PROTECTION FROM HARM

Risk management implies a sense of control over risk. It suggests that if we undertake the assessment properly and put appropriate strategies in place, then the risk will no longer be an issue. Firstly, this approach to life fails to recognise the uncertainty of risk and the inability to accurately predict exactly what is likely to happen and in what circumstances. Secondly, it starts from the belief that all risks should be managed.

Attempting to assess risk might be a very useful exercise in ensuring that people think carefully through the potential consequences of their actions. However, it is not as easy to accept that because a potential risk has been identified, it necessarily should be managed. Inevitably, concentration on risk identifies real risks but it is also likely to identify potential virtual risks that warrant no further action. The danger of risk assessment is that it inevitably leads us to move into trying to devise a plan for all risks identified, not just those that should be selected for our attention.

Risk management also runs the risk of paternalism and being too parental in relation to those in our care. Paternalism can, while meant well, be an abuse of power over those in care. Whilst it is clear that care workers do owe service users a duty of care, and this includes a duty to protect them from harm, it does not provide care workers with a licence to override others' wishes, beliefs and rights in the name of protection. Most of the service users in care, although they may be vulnerable, are perfectly capable and, in law, entitled, to make decisions about their own lives, including the risks that they wish to engage in. Care workers are expected to care, to support, to help, even to advise, but not to control. For those very vulnerable people who do not have the capacity to make risk choices, the same process of assessment should be worked through, with the care worker trying, where possible, to reflect the service user's known views and involving family and other care workers; although it is acknowledged that a greater level of protection might be desirable for those who are unable to express a preference.

The language of risk management is not well suited to the personal care of individuals because it causes us to take an unnecessarily negative approach to risk by assuming that risk management is only about prevention. If this is the interpretation, then risk management is best suited to the development of policy and systems at organisational level. Risk management is particularly well suited to the airline industry, for example, where failure to engage in risk management would have devastating consequences, and where the risk management itself results in relatively little inconvenience for passengers when compared with the increased safety that it offers. Of course, at organisational level in health and social care, risk management also fulfils an important role in protecting the public and promoting safety. However, the same cannot be said of the individual care environment where attention to risk and restriction of rights in relation to a potential harm may have a significant, negative impact on the individual.

Managed risk-taking

Titterton (2005) proposes a move away from risk management and towards a managed risk-taking approach in the individual care environment. This does not mean that risks should not be assessed and explored but, rather, that risks are approached from a more positive perspective. Given that it is impossible to eliminate risk, and given the positive outcomes of risk-taking, how can we enable the service user to engage in this risk, while appropriately protecting them from unnecessary harm? Titterton proposes a step approach to risk-taking.

- *Consult and communicate* – this involves an opportunity for all interested parties to discuss their point of view.
- *Prepare a risk plan* – which identifies who has been consulted, what has been decided, who is responsible, timescales and how risk will be monitored and outcomes measured. It also includes what records will be kept.
- *Sign up* – all interested parties should sign and agree a risk plan.
- *Share information* – all involved must be fully informed.
- *Monitor and review* – even the best laid plans may need reviewing.
- *Support staff* – when appropriate processes are in place and reasonable care has been taken, it is important that staff are supported, even if a negative outcome ensues. The point is not to blame but to try to find out why something happened, so that it can be anticipated in the future (Titterton, 2005, pp.93–5).

CONCLUSION

Independence and the ability to live life according to one's own preferences, beliefs and choices are important values in maintaining a good quality of life. Protecting an individual's right to independence is no less important than protecting an individual from harm. Consequently, it is important to teach practitioners how to support service users to engage in risk safely. Equally, organisations need to learn how to support practitioners in appropriate risk-taking with those in their care. Risk management and the promotion of independence should be a proactive activity. All too often it is reactive. We wait until something has happened and then we approach all other risks from a negative viewpoint. Either that or, because practitioners are frightened to take risks on behalf of their clients, they practise in a cautious and defensive manner. If, however, we address risk proactively, planned and positive risk-taking is a more likely outcome.

A welcome emphasis on user involvement, and the implementation of Expert Patient initiatives, demonstrate admirably that service users do not relish being 'told what to do in their best interests'. It is a salutary thought that the risks taken by service users are their risks not ours, and that to deny them choice in the decision-making process is probably foolhardy and is definitely arrogant. However, that does not mean that the practitioner has no responsibility for the actions or the outcome.

Protection from harm and the promotion of independence are not necessarily contradictory; unless they are interpreted as absolutes. If an individual must be protected from all possible harm, it is very unlikely that one would wish to allow any independence. Alternatively, promoting absolute independence in a care relationship is likely to lead to charges of negligence. As with many of the decisions in care, each situation must be assessed on its own individual merits and as much information, from a number of relevant sources, must be taken into account in the decision-making process. However, what is important to remember is how much each of us values our opportunities to be independent and to take risks, as well as our need, at times, to be protected. No less should be afforded to those in our care.

ACTIVITY 8.9

In partnership with a client (or friend, if you are not working in a care environment) undertake a risk assessment for a particular activity and try to develop a risk plan that enables appropriate risk-taking.

CHAPTER SUMMARY

Two key points to take away from Chapter 8:

- Care is no longer solely focused on what is in the best interests of the service user purely in respect of health gain; instead, care must take account of a number of different factors:
  - the responsibility of practitioners for the safety and protection of those in their care who may be more than ordinarily vulnerable
  - the need to anticipate and protect people from harm while not compromising independence unduly
  - the duty of the practitioner to raise any concerns that they may have in respect of the care and treatment of patients and service users
  - the need to treat people differently and to respect their individual differences and preferences
  - the promotion of independence and avoidance of a focus on risk prevention that leads to cautious and restrictive care.
- Managed risk-taking is an essential part of the care decision-making process.

FURTHER READING

Care Quality Commission (CQC) (2010) *Guidance about compliance. Essential standards of quality and safety.* London: CQC.

DoE (2013) *Working Together to Safeguard Children: a guide to interagency working to safeguard and promote the welfare of children.* London: HM Government.

DH (2005a) *Independence, Wellbeing and Choice: our vision for the future of social care for adults in England.* London: Department of Health.

HMSO (2014a) *Care Act 2014*. London: The Stationery Office.

DH (2011) *Protection of Vulnerable Adults – principles of safeguarding*. London: HM Government.

Godin, P. (ed.) (2006) *Risk and Nursing Practice*. Basingstoke: Palgrave Macmillan.

Penhale, B. and Parker, J. (2008) *Working with Vulnerable Adults*. Abingdon: Routledge.

09

VALUES, ACCOUNTABILITY AND RESPONSIBILITY

LEARNING OUTCOMES:

In this chapter you will:

- Reflect on the practitioner's responsibility to provide good quality, up-to-date evidence-based care

- Identify appropriate professional and care standards derived from core values

- Examine accountability in practice; specifically relating to practitioners, care provider organisations and care regulators.

INTRODUCTION

The Francis Inquiry Report (2013) has placed the accountability of practitioners firmly back on the agenda. Important questions about the responsibility and accountability of practitioners were raised following the failings of staff at Mid-Staffordshire NHS Trust to meet expectations for good standards of care. Specifically, the Report cites the failure of staff to meet their responsibility to provide safe, compassionate and effective care, the failure of senior managers, the failure of the Board to protect patients and to ensure that care standards were met and the failure of inspectors and regulators to identify the problems and call practitioners and providers to account. This chapter will explore what it means to be responsible and accountable for care provision and articulates what actions must be taken when any incident or breach in respect of that care is found to have occurred.

Although expected standards of care are articulated by national and professional standards, the actual quality of care that is provided is determined by the values and standards and behaviours of individual practitioners and by the pervading values and culture within the organisation within which an individual practises. Values, as discussed in earlier chapters, are the beliefs and attitudes held by an individual and which should underpin the manner in which care will be given. Standards of care are agreed benchmarks against which individual care practice can be measured and monitored (e.g. either internally through a series of quality metrics; or externally through assessment from the Care Quality Commission, Monitor, SCIE, etc.). If care provision is found to be below the standards expected, practitioners are held responsible and may be called to account for their actions and when in responsible roles, for the actions of others. In order to be responsible and accountable for their actions practitioners need to understand both what they should be doing, and why they should be doing it. They must also be able to evaluate a situation and select appropriate behaviours and interventions and apply them appropriately to the individual context. Organisations are now bound by 'A Duty of Candour' (Health and Social Care Act amendment 2014) and this will be discussed later in the chapter.

Although practitioners rarely overtly discuss their underpinning values, it is true to say that values should be the fundamental determinants of the quality of care that the patient receives. Values underpinning care provision are frequently articulated on behalf of the care practitioner in a variety of different forms. These can be formal and legally binding expectations of values and standards of care, as expressed in professional codes of practice, national care standards, national service frameworks or care strategies, care pathways and law which formally articulate underpinning values and standards for care provision. Alternatively, standards can be a more informal expression of values and intentions as articulated in vision statements and philosophies of care.

ACTIVITY 9.1

Conduct a search to see how many different expressions of standards you can find that are relevant to your work area.

- Were you aware of the promises that have been made about the service you will be providing?

- Do you feel adequately prepared to provide that service?

Examples of places to look may be: the Department of Health website, The Care Quality Commission website, Skills for Health, Skills for Care and the websites of other relevant professional organisations and societies. You may also look in your workplace to see if there is a vision statement, expression of service standards or commitments to an expressed philosophy of care.

RESPONSIBILITY AND ACCOUNTABILITY IN PRACTICE

Providing care for others is different from work in other occupations because of its personal and intimate nature and because many of the recipients of care are 'more than ordinarily vulnerable' (Sellman, 2011, p.49). Care work cannot be viewed as 'just a job' in the way that it is possible to view working at the checkout in a supermarket. Unlike customers in a supermarket, patients and service users need to place their trust in another's hands. Unlike a supermarket, individuals in a care setting invite strangers to participate in the most private and intimate aspects of their lives. Also, unlike a supermarket, if patients do not like the service they receive they are frequently unable to take their business elsewhere. Care practitioners are in a very privileged, but also very responsible, position. It has been claimed that the way in which we treat the most vulnerable in society is a reflection of the values, ethics, compassion and standards of that society (Seedhouse, 2009). In order to protect the most vulnerable, and for society to fulfil its obligations to those that are most vulnerable, standards of practice are set. These standards are derived from the underlying beliefs and values about how we should treat our fellow humans.

When a practitioner agrees to provide care they enter into a 'contract' with a patient or service user. This 'contract', much like any other agreement between two parties, imposes a set of obligations on the service provider. It also imposes a special duty and responsibility towards the person receiving care which requires the caregiver to meet specified standards of service and behaviour.

Being responsible and accountable

Being responsible means that individuals undertaking a particular role are required to meet the expectations of that role; if these expectations are not met, the individual who should have fulfilled the expectations can be held responsible. Different roles entail different responsibilities. As a parent I am responsible for the wellbeing, support and development of my children. As a teacher I may be responsible for meeting the learning needs of my students. As a caregiver I am responsible for facilitating the health, wellbeing, care and, where possible, rehabilitation of those within my care. As a manager I am responsible for the culture of the workplace, the competence of staff and for the design and implementation of policies and procedures to ensure safe and effective service. As a manager I also share responsibility for the actions of the people who work within my organisation. Different roles bring different levels of responsibility. Our responsibilities are often linked to our grade of employment and are usually articulated in a job or role description on commencement of employment.

ACTIVITY **9.2**

Review your role/job description if you have one (if you do not have one, consider asking your employer to provide you with one)

- Does this describe your responsibilities?
- If a patient looked at your role description, would they understand what they could expect from you?

From a very early age we begin to understand responsibility and the implications of failing to live up to our responsibilities and others' expectations. For example, the school child learns their responsibilities in learning by attending classes, listening and engaging in activities and by undertaking homework and assessment. If the child fails to accept these responsibilities their learning will be compromised. However, although we must be mindful of our different responsibilities, it is also important to recognise the boundaries of these responsibilities; the child does not, for example, have to help other students, nor to design their own learning programme.

It is not until we reach the age of eighteen, when the law recognises us as adults, that we become fully, legally responsible. Our parents may be ultimately legally responsible for us until we reach the age of maturity, but it does not mean that the law condones irresponsible or unlawful behaviour before this time. As soon as a child can understand and make reasoned decisions, they may share responsibility for some of their actions. As adults we are normally deemed to be sufficiently capable of making decisions for ourselves, by ourselves, and we can, therefore, be held legally and morally responsible for the actions and consequences that arise from those decisions and actions. When we are held legally responsible we are also accountable. That means that we may be called upon to explain, or account for, our actions (or failure to act) to someone who has the right to ask. It is very difficult to disassociate responsibility and accountability, except in respect of personal decisions that only affect yourself. I may be responsible for myself but I am not required to account to myself for my actions (although it could be argued that this is the process that occurs in truly, effective, reflective practice). As a general rule if we are held formally responsible then we are also accountable to someone.

To whom am I responsible and accountable?

The service user/patient

When we enter into a care relationship with another person, as well as being responsible for ourselves we also take on some responsibility towards the person being cared for. This responsibility brings with it the requirement for particular standards of performance to be maintained. In the case of the care practitioner this responsibility is expressed in law as a 'duty of care'. The duty of care is owed to any person for whom you are caring in an occupational capacity. This duty applies to all activities undertaken by the care practitioner, whether it is complex surgery or simply assisting with washing an individual. This duty of care requires that any intervention undertaken by the practitioner must be done to 'an appropriate standard'. It can be argued, however, that an appropriate standard is a very vague term. This is partly because the environment of care is constantly changing and partly because it would be impossible to articulate standards for every element of care provision in every circumstance. Therefore, there has to be an element of interpretation in what the law means in relation to an 'appropriate standard'. It is more easily understood from a negative perspective. When care fails to meet the standards set, the failure may cause distress, harm, humiliation, fear, neglect or simply loss of trust, and the practitioner can be held responsible.

The law

The judgement of whether an action is appropriate or not is made by applying a common principle – i.e., practitioners will be judged by measuring their performance against the standard of the 'ordinary, competent practitioner' undertaking that same role. That is to say, if practice is called into question, the performance will be judged on the basis of the normal standards of behaviour expected of other practitioners in similar roles. The key words to note in this judgement are 'ordinary' and 'competent'. Practitioners are not measured against the standards of the very best practitioner, or against the latest techniques, but are judged against generally acceptable practice. This judgement recognises the fact that practitioners are human; that they cannot be expected to always deliver exemplary, best practice, at the forefront of the discipline. However, it also recognises that patients are entitled to generally good standards, and the judgement tries to balance these interests. There have been a number of care failures in recent years that have rightly attracted public outrage. In some of these cases practitioners have faced disciplinary and legal proceedings and some of those found guilty have been imprisoned. In each of these cases expectations were failed because the expected standards of care were not met, the law has been invoked and some restitution sought (although it is a salutary thought that in some of the instances restitution could not be achieved for the patients who were harmed).

Another requirement of the law in respect of care is that the practitioner must be 'competent' within their sphere of expertise, and within the expectations of their role. It is, therefore, a responsibility of employers to ensure that practitioners have the relevant training and education to equip them to undertake their role and that they accept the responsibility to engage effectively with the training to enable them to work proficiently. You may be aware of mandatory training registers which record attendance at training such as 'Moving and Handling'. It also means that educators and trainers must assess and sign off that the practitioners have met the minimum standards of safety and proficiency following any training that has been undertaken.

Agreement about what constitutes acceptable and competent practice changes as work practices, public expectations and knowledge develop. These developments in practice may be the result of research which generates new evidence; if accepted, this new evidence should influence and change practice – this is what is meant by the term 'evidence-based practice'. The expectation for evidence-based practice places a responsibility on the care practitioner to ensure that their knowledge and practice remains up to date. Not all practitioners are required to generate evidence, but they are required to be aware of new and best evidence in their area of expertise and to base their practices upon it.

A duty of care is not a licence to control others and make decisions for them about their care, decisions that they should be making for themselves (see *Chapter 6* on autonomy). Neither is the duty of care a requirement to undertake roles outside of one's sphere of expertise and experience. It must be understood that a responsibility to a patient may require the practitioner to pass aspects of, or all of, their care on to someone more appropriate if the needs are outside of the knowledge and experience of the original practitioner. Knowing one's limits and boundaries and understanding appropriate action to take are important aspects of responsibility.

Responsibility to the employer

Employees are responsible for ensuring that they understand, agree with and fulfil the employment obligations laid down in their contract of employment. This usually requires them to undertake a particular set of duties and fulfil a contracted number of hours in a role. In addition, the practitioner will be required to ensure that they act in accordance with the policies and procedures of that organisation. Failure to meet those expectations may require the practitioner to account for their actions to a manager or to a disciplinary hearing. It should be remembered that, while the employer should make expectations easily available, the worker is responsible for familiarising themselves with and fulfilling the requirements of those expectations. As with other situations, ignorance is no defence in law.

Responsibility for others

As practitioners become more experienced and become leaders and/or managers, they are likely to assume responsibility not only for their own actions, but also for the actions of others. In the same way that practitioners owe a duty of care and responsibility to patients, so too do they owe a duty and responsibility to those fellow workers for whose care they are also responsible. Managers are responsible for ensuring that other practitioners are appropriately prepared and trained for the tasks that they are being asked to undertake and that they are properly supervised and supported while fulfilling their roles. The principle is that individuals should not be placed in situations in which they are out of their depth or where they may pose a threat to themselves or others. There are no hard and fast rules about what this means in practice and each situation and each individual must be assessed independently. Before tasks are delegated to others the manager must be reasonably confident that the task is within the individual's scope of competence. It is also important to note that even though an individual has received training in a particular task, it cannot necessarily be assumed that they will be competent at performing that task. If they have had little opportunity to practise the task, they may not be competent. Checking by asking the individual, or observing them undertake the task for the first time, is a responsible way of assuring oneself of their competence. From time to time things will not go as planned and this is an unfortunate fact of life. If an issue does arise, the manager as well as the care practitioner must be able to account for the actions and the decisions that they have made. That is, they must be able to explain what they did and why they did it.

LEADERSHIP IN CARE

There is a great deal of emphasis placed on leadership in the current care arena. Good leadership is an essential component for high performing practice. Leadership can occur at any level of an organisation. The individual leader does not need to be a manager, but they do need to be able to inspire and lead others. Leaders are normally people who are knowledgeable, visionary, who ask questions about the world and propose solutions with a view to encouraging others to change behaviours to bring about improvements. For leaders to flourish it is important that there is a culture that encourages questioning and innovation, that supports individuals to implement change and to take ownership for change. Leadership is important because it asks people to think about how things could be, rather than to accept how things are, and then to plan a realistic way of achieving a vision of the future. It implies collaboration with others. Leaders cannot be leaders unless they can inspire followers to follow them. Leaders must be willing to take responsibility for their actions and must be accountable to those they seek to lead. Accepting the notion and expectation that all staff can be leaders promotes a culture of job satisfaction in which all staff can feel that they own their work. In this type of culture individuals will be inspired to reflect on their work and suggest new ways of doing things and take more personal responsibility. This must be a more productive way of enhancing work than leaving it to the manager to come up with all the ideas. A culture of 'distributed' or 'collective leadership' effectively supports the requirement for practitioners to be responsible not only for their own care practice but also for that of others. It enables anyone, no matter how junior, to note failures and poor practice and to not only raise and escalate concerns appropriately but also to offer solutions.

'Collective leadership cultures are characterised by all staff focusing on continual learning and, through this, on the improvement of patient care. It requires high levels of dialogue, debate and discussion to achieve shared understanding about quality problems and solutions.'

(West *et al.*, 2014, p.5)

Significant attention is focused on successful leadership as a key component of improving care standards in the NHS. The NHS Leadership Academy has developed a Healthcare Leadership Model entitled *The Nine Dimensions of Leadership Behaviour* (NHS Leadership Academy, 2013). The Healthcare Leadership Model (see inside the back cover) is a three-dimensional model, identifying essential leadership dimensions; each of the nine behaviours in the model is shown on a four-part scale articulating characteristics of different levels of achievement in that specific characteristic. The levels are: essential, proficient, strong and exemplary. Thus, the model allows you to reflect and plot your own position on the scale for each leadership behaviour; for example, it is possible to be proficient in some and exemplary in others. The behaviours are not role related and can apply to anyone at any level in an organisation. The purpose of this model is to assist individuals and managers through appraisal to identify personal strength and areas for improvement to ensure that people maximise their potential.

The Nine Dimensions of Leadership

- **Inspiring shared purpose** is at the heart of the model.

  This requires leaders to value a service ethos, to be curious about how to improve services and patient care and to behave in a way that reflects the principles and values of the NHS.

  This is surrounded by other essential behaviours:
  - leading with care – having essential personal qualities to care, understanding unique qualities and needs of a team, providing a safe environment to enable others to do their job effectively
  - evaluating information – seeking out varied information, using information to generate new ideas and make effective plans for improvement and change, making evidence-based decisions that respect different perspectives and meet service user needs
  - connecting our service – understanding how health and social care services fit together and how different people, teams or organisations interact
  - sharing the vision – communicating a compelling and credible vision of the future in a way that makes it feel achievable and exciting
  - engaging the team – involving individuals and demonstrating that their contributions and ideas are valued and important for delivering outcomes and improvements

- holding to account – agreeing clear performance goals and quality indicators, supporting individuals and teams to take responsibility for results, and providing balanced feedback
- developing capability – building capability to enable people to meet future challenges, using a range of experiences as a vehicle for organisational learning, acting as a role model for personal development
- influencing for results – deciding how to have an influence on other people, building relationships to recognise others' passions and concerns; using interpersonal and organisational understanding to persuade and build collaboration.

(NHS Leadership Academy, 2013)

ACTIVITY 9.4

Access the NHS Leadership Academy Model via the Resources tab on the following website: leadershipacademy.nhs.uk/

Use the Model to assess your own personal capabilities and competencies for leadership.

RESPONSIBILITY AND THE EMPLOYER

The employer holds responsibilities in the care environment, both to the patients and their relatives and to the care practitioners employed by them. Employers are responsible for ensuring that care provision can be conducted in a safe environment and that appropriate equipment is provided to undertake the job safely and effectively. The employer is also responsible for ensuring that the employees have access to appropriate training and development in order to perform their role. Through employment the employer assumes vicarious responsibility for the actions of the employee. If, therefore, an employee is negligent or causes harm to an individual in their care, the employer will be held responsible and accountable for that harm, alongside the employee; and it is likely that the employer will incur any financial compensation costs that are awarded as a result of any harm, except in cases where the employee has been negligent or reckless. This does not absolve the employee of responsibility – they may be the subject of an internal disciplinary hearing or even a criminal prosecution if their actions are sufficiently serious or reckless.

ORGANISATIONAL RESPONSIBILITY AND ACCOUNTABILITY

In 2014 Regulation 20 was added to the requirements of the Health and Social Care Act of 2008. The regulation imposes a 'Duty of Candour' on health and social care organisations. This regulation is designed to ensure that providers are open and transparent with people who use services and other 'relevant persons' in relation to care and treatment. It also sets out some specific requirements that providers must follow when things go wrong with care and treatment, including informing people about the incident, providing reasonable support, providing truthful information and an apology when things go wrong. Providing health and social care carries with it the risk that from time to time things will go wrong or will not reach the standards required. The duty of candour requires that this is both acknowledged by providers and, more importantly, that action is taken to improve things. The duty of candour is intended to reassure the public that an organisation is acting in a safe and responsible way in maintaining and improving standards of care. It also acknowledges the public's right to know when an incident has occurred that affects them. The Care Quality Commission has a responsibility for inspecting care organisations and it sets out its responsibility in respect of the duty of candour in the following excerpt from its guidance documentation.

'In interpreting the regulation on the duty of candour we use the definitions of openness, transparency and candour used by Robert Francis in his report:
- Openness – enabling concerns and complaints to be raised freely without fear and questions asked to be answered.
- Transparency – allowing information about the truth about performance and outcomes to be shared with staff, patients, the public and regulators.
- Candour – any patient harmed by the provision of a healthcare service is informed of the fact and an appropriate remedy offered, regardless of whether a complaint has been made or a question asked about it'. (CQC, 2015).

For the practitioner this means that any failures, errors or lapses must be reported and investigated. This requirement also holds even when you are not directly involved. Each practitioner has a duty to raise any concerns they may have about standards of care; initially to their direct line manager but if this is not acted upon then concerns must be escalated through the appropriate channels. The Governing Board holds ultimate responsibility for standards and public safety and must be confident that concerns are raised and acted upon appropriately. Many organisations have flow diagrams to illustrate the process for raising concerns.

RESPONSIBILITY FOR THE MANNER IN WHICH CARE IS PROVIDED

While the practitioner has a legal responsibility to provide competent care (that is, they know what to do and can demonstrate that they are able to do it) most care practitioners will also have a responsibility to provide care in a particular manner. It is easy to teach someone to do a task competently. In fact, robots could be programmed to undertake some tasks competently. The fact that a task has been performed competently is a necessary condition for care, but it is not, however, sufficient. Care is a social interaction, not a mechanical task. For the person receiving the care, the experience of care is of equal importance to the fact that care has been provided competently.

ACTIVITY 9.5

Discussion

Imagine that you are in hospital waiting to have surgery. You have spoken to the surgeon who was very knowledgeable and who told you all the technicalities and potential risks of the operation. You also saw the anaesthetist who has explained her role and you have had routine pre-operative tests. The nurse has explained that you will be unable to eat and drink prior to the surgery. You will be taken to the theatre at 11 o'clock and will return to the ward once you are sufficiently awake, and your physiological signs will be closely monitored. They have all asked you whether you have understood what is going to happen. You have had your vital signs observations recorded, and you have signed a consent form. You have been safely prepared for theatre and are aware of what to expect. In the middle of the night you wake up scared about the impending surgery. You call the nurse who stands by you and repeats exactly everything that you have been told during the day. Having finished, she walks away to attend to someone else.

- Do you think that the nurse has provided care?
- What else could the nurse have done to provide you with better care?

It seems clear that the professionals providing the care in this case have done that which is technically required of them in relation to competent care. However, as a patient it would be easy to feel let down if this had happened to me. Care that is only based on competence and technical information fails to acknowledge the importance of the other essential component, the values base of care and the responsibility of treating me as a fellow human. The nurse could have acted differently, sat down and held the individual's hand and acknowledged their right to be afraid. He/she may have encouraged the patient to talk about their fears and acknowledge that they are real to the person. He/she may even have sought to provide evidence that their fears were likely to be unfounded. The practitioner may have done nothing more than sit with them and provided support. However, by being empathetic and acting appropriately in response to that empathy the nurse would have provided compassionate care. The care did not require action, it merely required 'being with someone'. Their fears about the forthcoming surgery may not be any less after the interaction, particularly as the nurse could not change the fact that the individual was still going to undergo surgery, but the patient may have a much more positive view of their experience following reassurance and kindness. Compassionate care may make a significant difference to how the individual approaches their surgery and how the individual recovers from it. Competence is, of course, a very important aspect of care provision, but the inclusion of compassion through values lifts the care provided from good care to that which is exceptional and memorable.

Some unpublished research with a service user and carer group asked them to identify what the attributes of a good care practitioner are. These were the features they identified, with competence coming well down in terms of importance:

- Kind and compassionate
- Loyal and dependable
- Honest
- Common sense
- Positive attitude
- Able to put the patient first
- Willingness to help
- Competence
- Self-motivated.

(Quallington, 2011)

PROFESSIONAL ACCOUNTABILITY AND CODES OF PRACTICE

The values that are evident in care are often not legal responsibilities but 'professional' responsibilities. These values are articulated in codes of practice. These codes set out the standards and expectations of different groups of practitioners and seek to articulate the specific beliefs and practices that the public can expect when in contact with that group. When we fail to meet the value standards of our 'professional' group, individuals have a right to report us to the organisations that regulate practice.

Codes of practice provide practitioners with broad principles to guide their actions and behaviours. However, they cannot be used as a rulebook to tell practitioners what to do in every situation. Although codes of practice have an important role in guiding practitioner behaviours, they have also been criticised because of the ambiguity that they can create when two or more of the guiding principles expressed in the codes conflict (Wainwright and Pattison, 2004).

ACTIVITY 9.6

With a colleague, reflect on a Code of Practice and try to identify any conflicting principles.

Discuss what practitioners can do when faced with apparently conflicting guiding principles.

If a regulatory body is alerted that an individual has breached the code of practice, an investigation will occur and the practitioner may be called to account for their actions at a hearing. Such a hearing carries no weight in law but may adversely impact on the individual's specific role or rights to work in that kind of employment. If the complaint is sufficiently serious it could result in prosecution as well. For example, if a care worker is accused of hitting someone in their care, they would be in breach of a code of practice but would also be at risk of prosecution for assault. In care practice we have a responsibility to and for service users, to our employers to ensure that we fulfil the requirements of our role, to the law and we may also have a responsibility to a regulatory body. Wherever it can be demonstrated that we have a responsibility, we may be called to account for our actions in relation to that responsibility. That is, we may be asked to justify what we have done and why we have done it.

When called to account, there are several ways that this account can be given. This is sometimes in person at an interview or by giving formal evidence. However, this could be in other forms such as production of care records or a formal written statement of events. Accurate record-keeping is therefore of vital importance in evidencing care provision and underlying values.

MAINTAINING RECORDS

The maintenance of accurate and contemporary records plays an important role in ensuring consistent, planned care and the appropriate review and assessment of care. However, records may also be used to account for your practice. In spite of the important role that record-keeping plays in care provision, it is often seen as a burdensome chore and it is well documented that it is an activity that is done badly (Dimond, 2005; Reid, 2005). Reviews of records in social care (Trevithick, 2005) have criticised records for:

- failing to record baseline information
- failure to note deterioration or improvement of condition
- failure to record decisions or conversations
- failure to link information together
- failure to provide indications of future care and intervention.

Looking at this list, one could be forgiven for wondering what role records are fulfilling. Perhaps it is because records are seen as an irksome activity that gets in the way of the real job of caring, that they are so badly kept. However, it cannot be stressed too much that accurate and careful record-keeping is for the good and protection of the care worker as well as the service user.

Hopefully you ticked all or nearly all of the above, as they all have a role to play in the maintenance of records.

There is a tension in record-keeping between recording sufficient accurate information and maintaining a succinct and manageable record (Prideaux, 2011).

Look at this list of the purposes of records and tick the ones you think are relevant:

- a legal requirement
- as a story about the client's care
- as a means of communication between different practitioners
- a report to document improvements, deteriorations, deviations from plans
- a record for goals and action plans
- as a means of documenting a client's express wishes
- as a means of ensuring consistency of care
- as a legal record of care and the treatment provided
- to record interactions with clients and family
- to protect the practitioner from claims that they did not provide good care
- as a historical record.

Coulshed and Orme (1998) state that records should record: 'significant facts, evidence, feelings, decisions, action taken, planned action and when actions should be monitored and reviewed'. One could add: tests undertaken; results received and significant conversations with clients or relevant others. Ensuring the accuracy of information in records is essential. Practitioners should avoid recording value judgements and hearsay and should avoid statements that do not convey any useful information such as, for example, 'usual care given' or 'needs assistance with walking'. If a practitioner was asked at a later date to account for what that meant specifically, they would probably be unable to remember the specifics of that particular person's care. It is much better to briefly note what was actually done for the individual and what specific assistance is needed. It is a salutary lesson to stop and think 'If I am asked about this in five years' time in a court of law, will I know what I meant?' 'Will there be enough information in my records to help me remember the specific care that was given to that particular person and the reasons for the care that was provided?' The maxim that is often used to remind practitioners of the importance of records is: 'If it hasn't been recorded then it hasn't happened'.

An increasingly common method of validating records is, where possible, to do this in partnership with service users and patients. As a nurse it often used to frustrate me to read in the notes that the person had 'slept well' only to be told by the patient, 'I had such a bad night, nurse'. Service users are keen to be involved in their care and, while it may take more time, it is likely to improve the accuracy of the records written and the appropriateness of the interventions planned.

Statements as an account of practice

Formal statements may be used as a legal document to assess what happened at an event or to make a judgement about the quality and circumstances of someone's care. Statements should be used as a means of recording a factual account of events to the best of your knowledge. Detail is important, but only relevant detail. Statements should not be used as an opportunity to suggest who else could be to blame or to pass opinions on others' behaviours and actions. Neither are they an opportunity to write a story.

ACTIVITY   9.8

- Read the statement in *Figure 9.1* and underline the facts of the case in one colour. Then, in another colour, underline anything that you think is hearsay or assumption or irrelevant material.
- Rewrite the statement as a factual account of events.
- Reflect on the values and actions of the care assistant expressed in this statement and think about how the values expressed influenced the unfortunate outcome of the situation. How should the care assistant have acted?

Saturday 24th May 2007. The nurse, Julie Brown, came on duty as usual at 7.45, even though she was due on duty at 7.30. I think she had difficulty getting out of bed, but nobody seemed to bother, it's not fair, everyone else has to get to the ward on time. Anyway, because she is late it always makes it late when medicines are given out and I expect that on this morning she had to rush to get things done. Nurse Brown gave the medicines out as usual and then we, the care assistants, had to do the washes. We always have to do the boring jobs. I was asked to help Florence with her wash. My heart sank. I find her difficult to cope with because she always asks questions about everything you do. When I got there she asked me, if the water was hot? Had I got her clean clothes? She didn't want the green cardigan I had got out, but wanted me to change it for the red one, I've been looking after her long enough, I know what she likes. She is lucky that anyone does anything for her! Half way through the wash she asked me why Nurse Brown had given her different pills today. I told her that the nurse knows what she is doing and that the doctor had probably changed her prescription. I asked if she had taken her pills, but she said that she hadn't because she did not know what they were. I said that they must be right if the nurse had given them to her and I stood by her while she took them. Later on the nurse called me into the office and said that Florence had been given the wrong pills and that I had to write a statement. It's not my fault that she took the wrong pills. I am not responsible for giving patients their pills. That nurse should have checked more carefully.

Figure 9.1 *A medication error.*

The statement has been used, by the care worker, as a platform to complain about her role, complain about a patient and complain about her colleagues and their actions, even though all of this is opinion and outside the responsibilities of her role. She has recounted the actual facts of the situation but these are hidden among lots of subjective statements and conjecture. She attempts to push the responsibility of her actions on to the nurse, who may have made an initial error in giving the wrong tablets; however, the error was then compounded by the care worker who overrode the concerns of the patient. The statement is a clear expression of the care worker's values. She fails to respect service users, she clearly sees individual care as burdensome and she abuses her position as a care worker to control the actions of those in her care. However, while assuming a position of power in relation to the patient, she is reluctant to assume that responsibility when called to account and fails to recognise her own responsibility in relation to the drug error.

CONCLUSION

Practitioners are required to make endless decisions in their day-to-day work. The decisions they face are often not easy and there are frequently no absolute rules about how to act. Care work is a responsible activity and, in fulfilling that responsibility, care workers need to be guided by core care values, codes of practice and standards of care, all of which articulate the expectations that should be met. It is also a fact that care workers will be called to account for what they have done and, at times, for what they have failed to do. Responsibility and accountability are, of necessity, indivisible.

Accountability is an essential component of the protection of the public. However, accountability serves another purpose; it is a mechanism through which practice can be monitored, reflected upon and, where necessary, improvements can be made. Practitioners are responsible to those in their care, their employers and sometimes their regulatory body. They are required by law to fulfil their duty of care to service users and their carers. Practitioners may be called to account for their actions informally or formally, either in person or through written records or formal statements.

Good record-keeping is essential in ensuring that the practitioner is able to communicate effectively to others and to provide evidence that will assist the practitioner to be able to recollect actual care provided and account for their actions.

The essential component of good, quality care is the need to ground all care within the care value base and to understand that how we do something is just as important as what we do. If values remain at the heart of practice then care will not only be competent but will also be respectful, caring and compassionate, and responsibility and accountability will not be such frightening concepts.

CHAPTER SUMMARY

Three key points to take away from Chapter 9:

- Care work requires practitioners to be responsible for both their actions and their failures to act when they should have done. When you assume responsibilities you may be called to account if these responsibilities are not met.
- Good leadership is an essential component for high performing practice; leadership can occur at any level of an organisation.
- It is imperative to maintaining current, accurate, factual and concise records.

FURTHER READING

Audit Commission (1995) *Setting the Records Straight.* London: Audit Commission.

CQC (2015) *Regulation 20: Duty of candour Information for all providers: NHS bodies, adult social care, primary medical and dental care, and independent healthcare.* London: CQC.

HSC Annual Report. London: Health Service Commissioner.

NHS Leadership Academy (2013) *The Nine Dimensions of Leadership Behaviour.* Leeds: NHS Leadership Academy.

NMC (2015) *The Code: professional standards of practice and behaviour for nurses and midwives.* London: NMC.

NMC (2013, updated 2015) *Guidance on Raising Concerns.* London: NMC.

NMC/GMC (2014) *Joint Guidance on Duty of Candour.* London: NMC.

Prideaux, A. (2011) Issues in nursing documentation and record-keeping practice. *British Journal of Nursing,* **20(22):** 1450.

West, M., Eckert, R., Steward, K., and Pasmore, B. (2014) *Developing Collective Leadership for Health Care.* London: King's Fund.

10

CONCLUSION: VALUE-BASED REFLECTION

THE ROLE OF VALUES

Positioning values centre stage in care practice will help practitioners to recognise and to deliver good care. In this book we have focused on the key values that we consider to be essential to good care practice. As has been discussed, caring has a qualitative dimension as well as a competency dimension. The quality of the care interaction determines how the recipient experiences care; providing good care demands something more from the practitioner than simply performing a task, no matter how competently the task is done. This qualitative dimension is guidance about the way in which care should be carried out. The chapters in this book have explored the concept of care and reflected upon values and behaviours that underpin good, compassionate care. Many individuals in receipt of care experience vulnerability, either by virtue of illness, age, disability, pain or loss of confidence. As has been claimed, the way a society treats its most vulnerable is a measure of the moral character of that society (Seedhouse, 1998). As a society there is a strong belief in the provision of state-funded intervention, but if it is to remain a valuable asset the quality of that care must be consistently good. We have claimed in this book that values are an essential component of good, moral care practice.

The merit of a set of articulated values has been discussed elsewhere in the book but, in summary, values:
- set acceptable, good standards of behaviour
- provide a guide for practitioners against which they can reflect and then develop and deliver good care
- provide a benchmark for others to judge standards of care.

However, it should be noted that while agreed values provide a guide for practitioner behaviour, they are not a set of rules. At times values will conflict and, sometimes, they will conflict with the beliefs, values or judgements of service users and of other practitioners. At times, you will need to understand how to determine the primacy of values and to whom they are owed, in order for you to disentangle them to make good decisions.

This book explores values in care and discusses the origins and relevance of these values and their application to care practice.

The activities in this book have been devised to enable you to explore your own values and practice and to reflect on these in the light of the expressed values underpinning care practice. Think about what you have learned about yourself and about others from participating in the activities in this book. It is true to say that you will face value-based challenges for as long as you practise. In fact, it would be worrying if you did not, as this might indicate that your practice was routinised and unresponsive to individual needs and situations. This chapter will briefly summarise the values that have been addressed in this book, before looking to the future and asking how you can ensure that values are fully integrated into your care practice.

COMPASSION AND CARE

High profile failures in care have emphasised the need to return to the fundamental values of compassion and caring and place these centre stage in current policy and practice. *Chapter 3* sets out to explore the moral relevance of compassion and its relationship with the notion of 'good care'. It identifies caring as a virtue and considers what it means to have a moral attitude of caring behaviour. We acknowledge the value of compassion as being one necessary (if not solely sufficient) component of good care.

Compassion is a virtuous attitude and morally significant emotional response to another's suffering but it is not the only important value to be considered in the care relationship, as this book demonstrates. However, a combination of respect for humanity and a person's dignity, intelligent kindness and compassion provides a sound starting point for good care and reflects the views of patients and service users. Good, compassionate care is more often experienced than understood intellectually and the mantra 'Do as you would be done by' should remind you to put yourself in that person's shoes and to think about what it is like and how it feels to experience care from another. This is as relevant to the small, everyday interactions of care as the more complex, demanding scenarios. Compassionate caring attitudes and behaviours can reduce suffering and have a positive impact on an individual's wellbeing. A range of exercises aim to help you to establish a shared definition and understanding of the moral value of compassion, and then to identify what is meant by good compassionate care and how this can be promoted in your care practice.

RIGHTS, EQUALITY AND ANTI-DISCRIMINATORY PRACTICE

Chapter 4 is important in setting the context for much of the care practice in today's health and care system. The language of rights or entitlements provides legitimacy for individuals to seek the kind of care that they need or desire. However, any claims fostered through a rights rhetoric must also recognise attendant responsibilities. This is particularly relevant in today's healthcare context which sees personal responsibility in respect of self-health-promoting behaviours by the population as a key element of a national healthcare system, the *NHS Five Year Forward View* (NHS, 2014).

Charters of rights are published by different groups to articulate their expectations and to provide a vehicle for challenging care when these expectations are not met. Generally, the rights that are articulated and claimed, particularly in the care context, are claims on another person or authority to provide the thing claimed. This is often the problem with a purely rights-based approach. Such an approach does not really help the practitioner who is faced by a rights claim but who may not have the resources available to meet the claim. Nor does this approach to care help the practitioner to adjudicate between competing claims. For example, if there were two people in equal need of a wheelchair, but only one wheelchair, how would the practitioner decide whose right it is to have their need met? However, in spite of these obvious difficulties, the publication and assertion of rights are very useful in both articulating entitlements and expectations, and for providing a vehicle through which care shortcomings can be challenged.

Rights rhetoric has also been the most influential factor in ensuring that more equal and fair treatment is available for those who have been unable to make their voice heard in other ways. Legislation to address issues around equality and various types of discrimination has been an essential component in raising awareness and making fairer opportunities for those in marginalised and discriminated groups. It is a shameful fact that discriminatory behaviour is still alive and well and is still widely perpetrated in the care environment. A focus on rights means that this is gradually improving and provides a platform to challenge and, where appropriate, prosecute anyone who persists in discriminatory behaviour.

RESPECT, DIGNITY AND AUTONOMY

It is, perhaps, a sad reflection on the way that others are treated that a 'rights rhetoric' is necessary. If all people were afforded the respect that they were due, by virtue of being a person, irrespective of age, sex, ability, colour or race, there should be no need to resort to claims for rights. *Chapters 5* and *6* demonstrate that respect is a fundamental value in care practice. Understanding respect for persons is a core value and, if this is properly understood and integrated into care, many of the other values will flow from it. Respect for persons in care facilitates the partnership philosophy of care that promotes dignity for clients even in situations of great dependence.

Being respected, having our views taken seriously, being able to express our individuality, being able to make, and act on, our own decisions and choices, and being able to devise our own goals, are very prized features of our everyday lives. It is these things that give us a sense of worth and a sense of self. It follows, then, that if these things are important to us, they are also of equal importance to those for whom we provide care. *Chapters 5* and *6* explored the notion and extent of respect and examined the duties of the care practitioner in ensuring that these values underpin practice. The activities in these chapters provided you with an opportunity to examine your own approach to care and to think about strategies that would enable you to enhance respect and dignity and provide opportunities to support those in your care to be autonomous.

TRUST, CONFIDENTIALITY AND TRUTH-TELLING

Chapter 7 identified that all caring and therapeutic relationships need to be established on the foundation of trust. Care recipients trust practitioners to act in their best interests, to be knowledgeable, to be caring in their approach and to do them no harm. Practitioners trust clients to be honest and to work in partnership with them. The notion of trust is important in any relationship. However, it is even more important in the care relationship where the service user puts themself in another's hands, often a complete stranger, and then allows them access to the most private and intimate aspects of their lives, both physical and emotional. In such situations the practitioner is very privileged and carries a huge responsibility to respect that trust placed in them and to take the responsibility of the caring role very seriously.

In order to care effectively it is also frequently necessary to know information about others to which one is not normally privy. In view of this, the care practitioner is trusted, through the principle of confidentiality, to keep the information they are entrusted with safe. This is not always an easy and clear-cut activity and the appropriate sharing of information can be very confusing and challenging. The section on confidentiality provided you with an opportunity to explore the nature, limits and potential exceptions to the rule of confidentiality. In addition, this chapter explored the concept of truth and the notion of truth-telling as a fundamental feature of trust in the care relationship.

PROTECTION FROM HARM AND PROMOTING INDEPENDENCE

At times a service user cannot or does not want to be autonomous, or sometimes expectations are placed on us by others which suggest that keeping a client safe and protecting from harm is in the client's best interests. While protection from harm and a client's best interests are often at opposite ends of the spectrum, it is not true that they always are so. *Chapter 8* recognised the responsibility that practitioners have in protecting those in their care from harm. However, the chapter tried to do this from the 'respect for persons' perspective. In contemporary care protection from harm and risk management have become dominant considerations in care, and are frequently the motivating factor for care decisions. *Chapter 8* argued that, although these are obviously important, they cannot be the only considerations on which care is based. While we must act in the client's best interests, it might be argued that best interests are not always served by being overly protective.

The chapter argued that risk is an essential, and often enjoyable, feature of all our lives. Taking risks can enhance our lives. Even when risk-taking goes wrong, we gain valuable learning and this contributes to our personal development. The tension for the care practitioner is to try to establish what risks are acceptable and what responsibilities they hold towards those in their care, in terms of protecting them from harm. The chapter provided a model for managed risk-taking, which provides the practitioner with a framework for considering risks, in discussion, where possible, with the service user and other relevant parties, and provides practitioners with evidence of that consideration.

VALUES, ACCOUNTABILITY AND RESPONSIBILITY

Chapter 9 explored the relationship between values and the notions of accountability and responsibility. This chapter identified that if you engage in a care interaction with another, you are responsible for ensuring your capability to undertake care and you are also responsible for the standard of your care provision. You are also accountable for your actions and you may be asked to explain your actions to anyone who has a right to ask; this could be the client, the employer, a professional or regulatory body, or the law. It is therefore important to understand what you are doing and why you are doing it, and not to undertake activities that are beyond the scope of your capability. Standards of care and codes of practice have been devised to provide a guide for practitioners and protection for clients. It is your responsibility to be aware of the standards and codes that relate to your own area of practice and to reflect on your practice in the light of these expectations.

Another important aspect of accountability is the records that are kept in respect of care provided. Records should provide evidence of actual care given. It is important that they are factual, informative and clear; they should note any changes in the service user's condition or situation and any significant conversation with that individual, their relatives or other practitioners. Records should not contain judgemental statements, hearsay or vague statements. Records provide a platform from which other practitioners can plan further care. Records also enable practitioners to assess a service user's progress or deterioration. If you are ever called to account for your actions, your records will be used to provide evidence of the care you provided.

WHERE TO NEXT?

This book has argued that understanding and integrating values as core elements of care practice is an essential to deliver good care. So now you have read the book and explored these key values, what do you do with the information and how do you know that you have been successful in centralising values into your practice?

Reading a book on values will not necessarily provide you with a prescription to solve the next difficult situation that you encounter in practice. This book provides you with knowledge about why a value is important, which values are important in the care context and what the tensions might be in adopting a value, and provides you with some examples of how values can be integrated into your practice. The next step is for you to take. Nobody's practice will ever change or improve if they always do what they have always done, in the way that they have always done it.

VALUES-LED REFLECTION

It is our belief that concentrating on values, that is to say, being confident about the desired beliefs and behaviours that underpin good practice, understanding how and why you do what you do, is the most important means of improving your practice. We recommend that 'values-led reflection' is an important skill to learn. Reflective practice is well accepted and expected in the care environment; there are a number of different models that can be used to assist the practitioner, for example, Kolb (1984), Rolfe (2001) and Oelofsen (2012). Reflective practice requires a practitioner to think about their practice and examine what they do in the light of theory and evidence. In addition, it offers the opportunity to change practice or to justify to themselves and others that they have acted appropriately. 'Values-led reflection' uses the same skills but requires the practitioner to use values as the focus for their reflection.

Reflecting on values provides you with an opportunity to analyse your own values base and examine the care you provide to your patients in the light of the care you would like to provide in an optimum circumstance. In addition, values-led reflection helps you to think through a rationale for care and to think about strategies to overcome barriers to providing values-led care. Reflective practice is often interpreted as reflecting on critical or dramatic incidents in order to see if the situation could have been managed differently. We suggest that values-led reflection is most valuable when it is used to explore and analyse aspects of everyday care; things that become so routine and second nature to the practitioner that they are no longer consciously aware of how or why they do them in the way that they do. This approach helps to guard against routinised behaviours that have become accepted practice but which might not always represent best practice. Hopefully, by learning to engage in values-led reflection, you will start to see what you do with 'new eyes', what Schön identifies as 'extraordinarily re-experiencing the ordinary' (Schön, 1987, p.93).

As discussed previously, there is no magic formula that outlines exactly how you must interact with patients to provide good care. How you do it will not necessarily be exactly the same as how a colleague may undertake the same activity. What is important is that your approach consistently reflects good values, professional standards and the needs, expectations and values of the care recipient. In addition, it is important that you can draw on a framework that enables you to account to others for your actions.

Reflective practice requires that you examine your practice and think about why you have acted in a particular way, and enables you to question the appropriateness or otherwise of that action.

Values-led reflection does not need to be done as an isolated activity. The exercise is just as valuable, possibly more so, when undertaken in a group. The added advantage is that when there are differences of understanding you have an opportunity to explore others' beliefs, values and interpretations and you will develop a better shared understanding of the factors that impact on your practice and that of others. Once you are confident about the dominant values that guide your own personal practice, you may choose to share this with those in your care. This is particularly helpful in preventing frustrations that may result from differences in expectations. If the patient/service user is under the impression that you, as the practitioner, will do everything for them, they will feel cheated and let down if your principal value is to facilitate independence.

The following are a series of statements that you can reflect upon to help you to engage in values-led reflection, and to help you identify your preferred personal values approach to practice.

- Care practice is a moral activity and values are as integral to good care delivery as are knowledge and skills.
- In order to provide values-led care it is necessary to reflect on and understand your own personal and professional values (those fundamental beliefs that will guide your attitudes and behaviours).
- Values-led reflection provides practitioners with a deeper understanding of the manner in which they wish to practise and provides a framework for assessing practice.
- Values-led reflection can empower the care practitioner as it provides a vehicle to challenge one's own practice and that of others.
- Values-led practice requires that practitioners take responsibility for the standards of care that they provide and requires that they reflect on the care that they see others provide and act on this where appropriate.

In reflecting on care from a values stance, there are a number of questions which you should reflect on:

1. What are the key values underpinning my care practice? (What do I believe about the nature of care and the duties I as a professional owe to those in my care?)
2. How integral are these values and philosophies to the care that I provide? (Always, sometime? Never?)

3. Which, if any, values am I prepared to compromise?
4. What compromises my ability to put my values into practice?
5. What strategies do I have to address these inhibitors?
6. How flexible is my practice in accommodating individual patient needs and how effectively do I work in partnership with those in my care?
7. Are my decisions and actions consistent and morally justifiable? (Could I account for and be comfortable with the reasons behind my actions, if called to do so?)
8. If I were giving this care again, what would I do differently? How would I have achieved this?
9. What do I need to do to enable me to provide care in the way that I would like?

Ethical values-led reflection can make a difference to the quality of patient care and the experience of care for the patient. Values-led reflection can also empower the professional to retain control of their own practice and assists them to deliver it in the manner that is consistent with their own professional values.

Reflecting on values and being more receptive to individual patient needs and preferences and integrating that into your practice will almost certainly guarantee that the patient will experience what they might describe as 'compassionate care'. That is to say, they will feel cared for. There is unlikely to be just one right way of doing things; most decisions are a matter of judgement (Johns and Freshwater, 2005). Professionals have choices about what they do and how they do it. Learning the language of values and recognising that all care interventions have a moral component should assist practitioners to deconstruct and reflect on practice and to determine best practice in any given situation; it will also assist in the articulation and justification of their practice and their decisions, both to others and to themselves.

Values-led reflection is only as good as the action that it leads us to. Therefore it is necessary to take reflection on from 'a looking back' exercise to 'a looking forward' exercise.

• Is there anything that I should do differently in respect of the care that I provide? (Think about specific examples.)
• Are there any different strategies that I can use to get round some of the barriers?
• Do I need any help to address these issues? If so, what would that help be?
• Is there anything about the care that others around me provide that I can learn from and integrate into my own practice?

The responsibility to raise concerns has received a very high profile in recent times. It is important that practitioners reflect on how they will manage this responsibility. No matter how junior you are, if you are feeling uncomfortable about another's practice it probably means that the issue would at least benefit from some exploration. There are a number of strategies available to you, depending on the severity of your discomfort. Here are just a few possible ways of raising concerns of others' practices. However, please remember that, if these are serious concerns, you are accountable for what you see and know, and you will be held responsible for making these concerns known to the appropriate manager or authority. Where you are unsure:

- You could adopt a genuinely interested stance and ask why someone does something in a particular way.
- You could ask another person if a particular action is acceptable practice or not (remember to maintain confidentiality).
- You could ask team members to engage in some shared reflective activities.
- You could look for evidence to illustrate that a particular practice is unacceptable and discuss it with the practitioner concerned.
- You could challenge the practitioner directly.
- You may feel the need to report your concerns to someone in a position of authority.

There is rarely a clear-cut answer to the question: 'Which strategy should I use?' Only you know your individual situation and circumstances. In addition, you need to consider the risks involved in engaging in any of the above strategies, but more importantly the risks of doing nothing. Do not forget that risks often pay off and have a positive outcome.

The purpose of value-led reflection is to help you to explore what kind of practitioner you want to be. It will help you to think about your practice in order to identify things that you can change in order to be more like the practitioner you want to be. Values-led reflection is not a once-only activity. It is a tool to be used again and again to check if you have developed bad habits or less good practice. Values-led reflection can also be used to help you decide what to do when you encounter new situations in care. Ultimately, it is hoped that it will improve practice. Values are at the core of good practice. If you invest time reflecting on your values and the ways in which they impact on your care, and you try to adapt your care where possible in the light of this reflection, it is likely that your care will be improved, bringing greater satisfaction to you and the care recipient.

FURTHER READING

Ghaye, T. (2000) *Reflection: principles and practice for health care professionals.* Dinton: Quay Books.

Johns, C. (2004) *Becoming a Reflective Practitioner.* Oxford: Blackwell.

Oelofsen, N. (2012) *Developing Reflective Practice.* Banbury: Lantern Publishing.

Tate, S. and Sills, M. (2006) *The Development of Critical Reflection in the Health Professions.* London: HEA.

REFERENCES

Alaszewski, A., Harrison, L. and Manthorpe, J. (eds) (1998) *Risk, Health and Welfare.* Buckingham: Open University Press.

Alderson, P. (2002) Young Children's Health Care Rights and Consent. *In* Franklin, B. (ed.) *The New Handbook of Children's Rights. Comparative policy and practice.* London: Routledge.

Alderson, P. (2000) *Young Children's Rights: exploring beliefs, principles and practice.* London: Jessica Kingsley Publishers.

Algase, D.L., Moore, D.H., Vandeweerd, C. and Gavin-Dreschnack, D.J. (2007) Mapping the maze of terms and definitions in dementia-related wandering. *Aging & Mental Health*, 11(6): 686–98.

Allen, A. (2011) *Unpopular Privacy: what must we hide?* New York: Oxford University Press.

Allen, A. (2011a) Privacy and Medicine, *The Stanford Encyclopedia of Philosophy* (Spring 2011 Edition), Edward N. Zalta (ed.). Available at http://plato.stanford.edu/archives/spr2011/entries/privacy-medicine/ (accessed 3 January 2017)

Almond, B. (1993) Rights. *In* Singer, P. (ed.) *A Companion to Ethics.* Oxford: Blackwell Publishing.

Alzheimer's Society (2013) *Safer Walking Technology Position Statement.* Available at www.alzheimers.org.uk/site/scripts/documents_info.php?documentID=579 (accessed 3 January 2017)

Armstrong, K. (2011) *Twelve Steps to a Compassionate Life.* London: The Bodley Head.

Association for Improvements in the Maternity Services (AIMS) (2012) Top Ten tips for what women want from their midwives. *Essentially MIDIRS*, 3(3): 27–31. Available at www.aims.org.uk/AIMSTopTenTips.pdf (accessed 22 January 2017)

Austin, W., Goble, E., Leier, B. and Byrne, P. (2009) Compassion Fatigue: the experience of nurses. *Ethics and Social Welfare*, 3(2): 195–214.

Aycock, N. and Boyle, D. (2009) Interventions to manage compassion fatigue in oncology nursing. *Clinical Journal of Oncology Nursing*, 13(2): 183–91.

Baier, A. (1986) Trust and antitrust. *Ethics*, 96: 231–60.

Baillie, L. (2007) *A case study of patient dignity in an acute hospital setting.* Unpublished thesis. London: London South Bank University.

Baillie, L. and Black, S. (2015) *Professional Values in Nursing.* London: CRC Press, Taylor and Francis Group.

Baillie, L., Gallagher, A. and Wainwright, P. (2008) *Defending Dignity. Challenges and opportunities for nursing*. London: RCN.

Ballatt, J. and Campling, P. (2011) *Intelligent Kindness: reforming the culture of healthcare*. London: RCPsych Publications, Royal College of Psychiatrists.

Banks, S. (2012) *Ethics and Values in Social Work*. 4th ed. Basingstoke: Palgrave.

Banks, S. and Gallagher, A. (2008) *Ethics in Professional Life. Virtues for health and social care*. Basingstoke: Palgrave Macmillan.

Bantry White, E. and Montgomery, P. (2014) Electronic tracking for people with dementia: an exploratory study of the ethical issues experienced by carers in making decisions about usage. *Dementia*, 13(2): 216–32.

Beach, M.C., Duggan, P.S., Cassel, C.K. and Geller, G. (2007) What does 'respect' mean? Exploring the moral obligation of health professionals to respect patients. *Journal of Society of General Internal Medicine*, 22: 692–5.

Beauchamp, T.L. (2007) The 'Four Principles' approach to health care ethics. *Chapter 1 in* Ashcroft, R.E., Dawson, A., Draper, H. and McMillan, J.R. (eds) *Principles of Health Care Ethics*. 2nd ed. London: John Wiley and Sons.

Beauchamp, T. and Childress, J. (2013) *Principles of Biomedical Ethics*. 7th ed. New York: Oxford University Press.

Beauchamp, T. and Childress, J. (2001) *Principles of Biomedical Ethics*. 5th ed. New York: Oxford University Press.

Beck, U. (1992) *Risk Society*. London: UCL Press.

Begley, A. (2010) On being a good nurse: reflections on the past and preparing for the future. *International Journal of Nursing Practice*, 16: 525–32.

Belcher, M. (2009) Graduate nurses' experiences of developing trust in the nurse–patient relationship. *Contemporary Nurse: a journal for the Australian nursing profession*, 31(2): 142–52.

Benner, P.B. (1984) *From Novice to Expert. Excellence and power in clinical nursing practice*. Menlo Park, CA: Addison-Wesley.

Beresford, P. (2013) *Beyond the Usual Suspects: towards inclusive user involvement: research report*. London: Shaping Our Lives.

Beyleveld, D. and Brownsword, R. (2001) *Human Dignity in Bioethics and Biolaw*. Oxford: Oxford University Press.

Bielby, P. (2005) The conflation of competence and capacity in English medical law: a philosophical critique. *Medicine, Health Care and Philosophy*, 8: 357–69.

Blum, L.A. (1987) Compassion. *In* Kruschwitz, R.B. and Roberts, R.C. (eds) *The Virtues: contemporary essays in moral character*. Belmont, CA: Wadsworth.

Blum, L.A. (1980) Compassion. *In* Rorty, A.O. (ed) *Explaining Emotions*. Berkeley, CA: University of California Press, pp. 507–17.

BMA (2009a) *Confidentiality and disclosure of health information tool kit*, 1st ed. London: BMA. Available at www.bma.org.uk/advice/employment/ethics/confidentiality-and-health-records (accessed 24 January 2017)

BMA (2009b) *Consent Tool Kit.* 5th ed. London: BMA.

Bondi, L., Carr, D., Clark, C. and Clegg, C. (2011) *Towards Professional Wisdom: practical deliberation in the people professions.* Farnham, Surrey: Ashgate Publishing Ltd.

Boore, J.R.P. (1978) *Prescription for Recovery: the effect of pre-operative preparation of surgical patients on post-operative stress, recovery and infection.* London: Royal College of Nursing (RCN research series).

British Association of Social Workers (2014) *The Code of Ethics for Social Work*, Birmingham: BASW.

Brooker, D. (2012) Understanding dementia and the person behind the diagnostic label. *International Journal of Person Centered Medicine*, 2(1): 11–17.

Brooker, D. (2007) *Person-centred Dementia Care: making services better.* London: Jessica Kingsley.

Brooker, D. (2003) What is person-centred care in dementia? *Reviews in Clinical Gerontology*, 13(3): 215–22.

Brooker, D. and Latham, I. (2015) *Person-centred Dementia Care. Making services better with the VIPS framework*, 2nd ed. London: Jessica Kingsley.

Brykczyńska, G. (1997) A brief overview of the epistemology of caring. *In* Brykczyńska, G. and Jolley, M. (eds) *Caring: the compassion and wisdom of nursing.* London: Arnold Hodder Headline.

Bubb, S. (2014) *Winterbourne View – Time for Change. Transforming the commissioning of services for people with learning disabilities and/or autism.* A report by the Transforming Care and Commissioning Steering Group, chaired by Sir Stephen Bubb. Available at www.england.nhs.uk/wp-content/uploads/2014/11/transforming-commissioning-services.pdf (accessed 3 January 2017)

Buchanan, A.E. and Brock, D.W. (1990) *Deciding for Others: the ethics of surrogate decision making* (Studies in Philosophy and Health Policy). Cambridge: Cambridge University Press.

Burnell, K.J., Selwood, A., Sullivan, T., *et al.* (2015) Involving service users in the development of the Support at Home: Interventions to Enhance Life in Dementia Carer Supporter Programme for family carers of people with dementia. *Health Expectations*, 18(1): 95–110.

Caldicott, F. (2013) *Information: to share or not to share? The Information Governance Review.* London: DH.

Calkin, S. (2011) Whistleblowing Mid Staffs nurse too scared to walk to car after shift, *Nursing Times. Net.* Available at www.nursingtimes.net/nursing-practice/specialisms/accident-and-emergency/whistleblowing-mid-staffs-nurse-too-scared-to-walk-to-car-after-shift/5036466.article (accessed 3 January 2017)

Cavendish, C. (2013) *The Cavendish Review. An independent review into healthcare assistants and support workers in the NHS and social care settings.* Available at www.gov.uk/government/uploads/system/uploads/attachment_data/file/236212/Cavendish_Review.pdf (accessed 3 January 2017)

Centre for Health Services Studies, British Geriatrics Society and Royal College of Physicians (2009) *Privacy and Dignity in Continence Care. Reflective guidelines for health and social care settings.*

Kent: University of Kent, Centre for Health Services Studies. Available at www.bgs.org.uk/pdf_cms/reference/privacy_in_continence_toolkit.pdf (accessed 3 January 2017)

Centre for Policy on Ageing (2009) Ageism and age discrimination in secondary health care in the United Kingdom. London: CPA.

Chochinov, J. (2007) Dignity and the essence of medicine: the A, B, C and D of dignity conserving care. *British Medical Journal*, 335: 184–7.

Christman, J. (2015) Autonomy in moral and political philosophy. *In* Zalta, E.N. (ed.) *The Stanford Encyclopedia of Philosophy* (Spring 2015 edition). Available at http://plato.stanford.edu/archives/spr2015/entries/autonomy-moral/ (accessed 3 January 2017)

Christman, J. (2004) Relational autonomy, liberal individualism, and the social constitution of selves. *Philosophical Studies*, 117: 143–64.

Clayton, J.M., Hancock, K., Parker, S., *et al.* (2008) Sustaining hope when communicating with terminally ill patients and their families: a systematic review. *Psycho-Oncology*, 17(7): 641–59.

Code, L. (1991) Second persons. In *What Can She Know? Feminist theory and the construction of knowledge*. Ithaca, New York: Cornell University Press.

Cole, C., Wellard, S. and Mummery, J. (2014) Problematising autonomy and advocacy in nursing. *Nursing Ethics*, 21(5): 576–82.

Commission on Dignity in Care for Older People (collaboration established by the NHS Confederation, the Local Government Association and Age UK) (2012) *Delivering Dignity. Securing dignity in care for older people in hospitals and care homes. Final report.* London: Local Government Association, the NHS Confederation and Age UK. Available at www.ageuk.org.uk/home-and-care/improving-dignity-in-care-consultation/ (accessed 3 January 2017)

Cotterell, P., Harlow, G., Morris, C., *et al.* (2010) Service user involvement in cancer care: the impact on service users. *Health Expectations*, 14: 159–69.

Coulshed, V. and Orme, J. (1998) *Social Work Practice: an introduction.* 3rd ed. Basingstoke: Macmillan BASW.

CQC (2015) *Regulation 20: Duty of candour information for all providers: NHS bodies, adult social care, primary medical and dental care, and independent healthcare.* London: CQC.

CQC (2014) *Southern Cross, Orchid View, September 2009 – October 2011. An analysis of the Care Quality Commission's responses to events at Orchid View identifying the key lessons for CQC and outlining its actions taken or planned.* London: CQC. Available at www.cqc.org.uk/sites/default/files/Orchid%20View%20Investigation%20Report.pdf (accessed 3 January 2017)

CQC (2013) *The State of Health Care and Adult Social Care in England in 2012/13*, HC 838. London: The Stationery Office.

CQC (2012) *The State of Health Care and Adult Social Care in England in 2011/12*, HC 763. London: The Stationery Office.

CQC (2011) *Dignity and Nutrition Inspection Programme. National Overview Report.* Newcastle upon Tyne: CQC.

CQC (2010) *Care Quality Commission: guidance about compliance. Essential standards of quality and safety.* London: CQC.

Crawford, P., Gilbert, P., Gilbert, J., Gale, C. and Harvey, K. (2013) The language of compassion in acute mental health care. *Qualitative Health Research*, 23(6): 719–27.

Crisp, R. (2008) Compassion and beyond. *Ethical Theory and Moral Practice*, 11: 233–46.

de Raeve, L. (2002) Trust and trustworthiness in nurse–patient relationships. *Nursing Philosophy*, 3: 152–62.

Denney, D. (2005) *Risk and Society.* London: Sage Publications.

Department for Constitutional Affairs (2007) *Mental Capacity Act 2005. Code of Practice.* Crown Copyright. London: The Stationery Office.

Department of Education (2014) *Promoting fundamental British values as part of SMSC in schools. Departmental advice for maintained schools.* London: DoE. Available at www.gov.uk/government/publications/promoting-fundamental-british-values-through-smsc (accessed 3 January 2017)

Department of Education (2013) *Working Together to Safeguard Children: a guide to interagency working to safeguard and promote the welfare of children.* London: HM Government.

Dewar, B. (2013) Cultivating compassionate care. *Nursing Standard*, 27(34): 48–55.

Dewar, B. (2011) *Caring about caring: an appreciative inquiry about compassionate relationship centred care.* Unpublished PhD thesis. Edinburgh: Edinburgh Napier University.

Dewar, B., Adamson, E., Smith, S., Surfleet, J. and King, L. (2014) Clarifying misconceptions about compassionate care. *Journal of Advanced Nursing*, 70(8): 1738–47.

Dewar, B. and Nolan, M. (2013) Caring about caring: developing a model to implement compassionate relationship-centred care in an older people care setting. *International Journal of Nursing Studies*, 50(9): 1247–58.

Dewar, B., Pullin, S. and Tocher, R. (2011) Valuing compassion through definition and measurement. *Journal of Nursing Management*, 17(9): 32–7.

Dewing, J. (2008) Personhood and dementia: revisiting Tom Kitwood's ideas. *International Journal of Older People Nursing*, 3: 3–13.

DH (2015) *Mental Health Act 1983: Code of Practice.* London: The Stationery Office. Available at www.gov.uk/government/publications/code-of-practice-mental-health-act-1983 (accessed 3 January 2017)

DH (2015a) *The NHS Constitution for England.* Updated 2015. London: DH. Available at www.gov.uk/government/publications/the-nhs-constitution-for-england (accessed 3 January 2017)

DH (2014) *Hard Truths. The Journey to Putting Patients First.* Volume 2 of the Government Response to the Mid Staffordshire NHS Foundation Trust Public Inquiry: Response to the Inquiry's Recommendations, Cm 8777-II, Jan 2014, London, The Stationery Office.

DH (2014a) *Requirements for registration with the Care Quality Commission. Response to consultations on fundamental standards, the Duty of Candour and the fit and proper persons requirement for directors.*

Available at www.gov.uk/government/uploads/system/uploads/attachment_data/file/327561/ Consultation_response.pdf (accessed 3 January 2017)

DH (2014b) *Requirements for registration with the Care Quality Commission. Annex A – Final regulations.* Available at www.gov.uk/government/uploads/system/uploads/attachment_data/file/ 327562/Annex_A.pdf (accessed 3 January 2017)

DH (2014c) Fundamental standards: improving quality and transparency in care. DH News 7th July 2014. Available at www.gov.uk/government/news/fundamental-standards-improving-quality-and-transparency-in-care (accessed 3 January 2017)

DH (2014d) *2014/15 Choice Framework.* London: DH. Available at www.gov.uk/government/ publications/nhs-choice-framework (accessed 3 January 2017)

DH (2014e) *Achieving better access to mental health services by 2020.* Available at www.gov.uk/ government/publications/mental-health-services-achieving-better-access-by-2020 (accessed 3 January 2017)

DH (2014f) *Care and Support Statutory Guidance.* Issued under the Care Act 2014. London, DH.

DH (2013a) *The NHS Constitution for England.* London: DH.

DH (2013b) *Winterbourne View. Transforming care: one year on.* London: DH.

DH (2013c) *Learning Disabilities – Good Practice Project.* London: DH. Available at www.gov.uk/ government/uploads/system/uploads/attachment_data/file/261896/Learning_Diasbilities_Good_ Practice_Project__Novemeber_2013_.pdf (accessed 3 January 2017)

DH (2013d) *Review of healthcare assistants and support workers in NHS and social care. 'The Cavendish Review'.* Independent report for the DH. Available at www.gov.uk/government/publications/review-of-healthcare-assistants-and-support-workers-in-nhs-and-social-care (accessed 3 January 2017)

DH (2013e) *To share or not to share? The Information Governance Review.* London: Department of Health.

DH (2012) *Interim Report: Winterbourne View* (review). London: Department of Health.

DH (2012a) *Caring for our future: reforming care and support.* Cm 8378. London: The Stationery Office.

DH (2012b) *Transforming Care: a national response to Winterbourne View Hospital. Department of Health Review Final Report.* London: Department of Health. Available at www.gov.uk/government/ uploads/system/uploads/attachment_data/file/213215/final-report.pdf (accessed 3 January 2017)

DH (2012c) *The Prime Minister's Challenge on Dementia.* London: Department of Health.

DH (2012d) *Winterbourne View Review. Good practice examples.* London: Department of Health. Available at www.gov.uk/government/uploads/system/uploads/attachment_data/file/213219/good-practice-examples.pdf (accessed 3 January 2017)

DH (2011) *Protection of Vulnerable Adults – principles of safeguarding.* London: HM Government.

DH (2011a) *No Health Without Mental Health: a cross-government mental health outcomes strategy for people of all ages.* London: Department of Health. Available at www.gov.uk/government/publications/ the-mental-health-strategy-for-england (accessed 3 January 2017)

DH (2010) *Healthy Lives, Healthy People: our strategy for public health in England*, CM7985. London: The Stationery Office.

DH (2010a) *Front Line Care: report by the Prime Ministers Commission on the future of nursing and midwifery in England*. London: The Stationery Office.

DH (2010b) *Essence of Care 2010. Benchmarks for the fundamental aspects of care*. London: The Stationery Office. Available at www.gov.uk/government/publications/essence-of-care-2010 (accessed 3 January 2017)

DH (2009) *Valuing People Now: a new three-year strategy for learning disabilities*. London: Department of Health.

DH (2009a) *Living Well with Dementia: a national dementia strategy. Putting people first*. London: Department of Health Publications.

DH (2009b) *Reference Guide to Consent for Examination or Treatment*, 2nd ed. London: Department of Health. Available at www.gov.uk/government/publications/reference-guide-to-consent-for-examination-or-treatment-second-edition (accessed 3 January 2017)

DH (2005a) *Independence, well-being and choice: our vision for the future of social care for adults in England*. London: The Stationery Office.

DH (2005b) *Research Governance Framework for Health and Social Care*, 2nd ed. London: The Stationery Office.

DH (2004a) *Choosing Health? Making healthier choices easier*. London: The Stationery Office.

DH (2004b) *Seeking consent: working with older people*. London: The Stationery Office.

DH (2001a) *National Service Framework for Older People*. London: The Stationery Office.

DH (2001b) *Valuing People: a new strategy for learning disability for the 21st century*, Cm 5086. London: The Stationery Office.

DH (1997) *The Caldicott Committee Report on the Review of Patient-Identifiable Information*. London: Department of Health.

DH and NHS Commissioning Board (2012c) *Compassion in Practice: nursing midwifery and care staff, our vision and strategy*. London: The Stationery Office. Available at www.england.nhs.uk/wp-content/uploads/2012/12/compassion-in-practice.pdf (accessed 3 January 2017)

DH and Poulter, D. (2013) *Treating patients and service users with respect, dignity and compassion*. Available at www.gov.uk/government/policies/treating-patients-and-service-users-with-respect-dignity-and-compassion (accessed 3 January 2017)

Dignity in Care (2015) *The Dignity Dos*. Available at www.dignityincare.org.uk/About/The_10_Point_Dignity_Challenge/ (accessed 3 January 2017)

Dillon, R.S. (2014) Respect, *The Stanford Encyclopedia of Philosophy* (Spring 2014 Edition), Edward N. Zalta (ed.). Available at http://plato.stanford.edu/archives/spr2014/entries/respect/ (accessed 3 January 2017)

Dimond, B. (2015) *Legal Aspects of Nursing*, 7th ed. Boston: Pearson.

Dimond, B. (2005) Exploring common deficiencies that occur in record keeping. *British Journal of Nursing,* 14(10): 568–70.

Dinç, L. and Gastmans, C. (2013) Trust in nurse–patient relationships: a literature review. *Nursing Ethics*, 20(5): 501–16.

Dinç, L. and Gastmans, C. (2012) Trust and trustworthiness in nursing: an argument based literature review. *Nursing Inquiry*, 19(3): 223–37.

Downie, R.S and Calman, K.C. (1994) *Healthy Respect. Ethics in health care.* 2nd ed. Oxford: Oxford University Press.

Downie, R.S. and Telfer, E. (1969) *Respect for Persons.* London: George Allen and Unwin.

Doyal, L. and Gough, I. (1991) *A Theory of Human Need.* Basingstoke: Macmillan.

Duggan, S., Blackman, T., Martyr, A. and Vanschaik, P. (2008) The impact of early dementia on outdoor life. A 'shrinking world'? *Dementia,* 7(2): 191–204.

Duncan, P. (2010) *Values, Ethics and Health Care.* London: Sage Publications.

Dworkin, G. (1988) *The Theory and Practice of Autonomy.* Cambridge: Cambridge University Press.

Edwards, S. (2009) *Nursing Ethics. A principle-based approach,* 2nd ed. Basingstoke: Palgrave Macmillan.

Elwyn, G. and Charles, C. (2009) Shared decision-making: from conceptual models to implementation in clinical practice. *In* Edwards, A. and Elwyn, G. (eds) *Shared Decision-making in Health Care: achieving evidence-based patient choice,* 2nd ed. Oxford: Oxford University Press.

Entwistle, V.A., Carter, S.M., Cribb, A. and McCaffery, K. (2010) Supporting patient autonomy: the importance of clinician–patient relationships. *Journal of General Internal Medicine,* 25(7): 741–5.

Equality and Human Rights Commission (2012) *Your Home Care and Human Rights.* London: Equality and Human Rights Commission.

European Nutrition for Health Alliance (2012) *Report from 'EU patient groups and the relevance of nutrition' conference 2012.* Available at www.european-nutrition.org/index.php/news/news_post/report_from_eu_patient_groups_and_the_relevance_of_nutrition_conference (accessed 22 February 2017)

Eyal, N. (2012) Informed consent. *In* Zalta, E.N. (ed.) *The Stanford Encyclopedia of Philosophy* (Fall 2012 Edition). Available at http://plato.stanford.edu/archives/fall2012/entries/informed-consent/ (accessed 4 January 2017)

Farsides, B. (2013) Consent and the capable adult patient. B: an ethical perspective – consent and patient autonomy. *In* Tingle, J. and Cribb, A. (eds) *Nursing Law and Ethics,* 4th ed. Oxford: Blackwell-Wiley, Ch. 7, pp. 151–65.

Farsides, C. (2005) How informed should consent be? *In* Webb, P. (ed) *Ethical Issues in Palliative Care.* Radcliffe Publishing Ltd.

Faust, H.S. (2009) Kindness, not compassion, in healthcare. *Cambridge Quarterly of Healthcare Ethics,* 18: 287–99.

Figley C. (ed.) (1995) *Compassion Fatigue. Coping with secondary traumatic stress disorder.* New York: Routledge Taylor & Francis Group.

Firth-Cozens, J. and Cornwell, J. (2009) *The Point of Care. Enabling compassionate care in acute hospital settings.* London: King's Fund.

Fletcher, J. (1972) Indicators of Humanhood: a tentative profile of man. *The Hastings Center Report*, 2(5): 1–4.

Flynn, M. (2012) South Gloucestershire Safeguarding Adults Board. *Winterbourne View Hospital – A Serious Case Review.* Liverpool: CPEA Ltd. Available at http://hosted.southglos.gov.uk/wv/report.pdf (accessed 17 February 2017)

Foot, C., Gilburt, H., Dunn, P., *et al.* (2014) *People in Control of their own Health and Care. The state of involvement.* London: King's Fund in Association with National Voices.

Francis, R. (2013) *The Mid Staffordshire NHS Foundation Trust Public Inquiry. Report of the Mid Staffordshire NHS Foundation Trust Public Inquiry.* February 2013, HC 898-III. London: The Stationery Office. Available at http://webarchive.nationalarchives.gov.uk/20150407084003/http://www.midstaffspublicinquiry.com/report (accessed 17 February 2017)

Francis, R. (2010) *The Mid Staffordshire Foundation NHS Trust Inquiry. Independent inquiry into care provided by Mid Staffordshire NHS Foundation Trust: January 2005 – March 2009. Volume I.* London: The Stationery Office.

Friedrichsen, M., Linholm, A. and Milberg, A. (2011) Experiences of truth disclosure in terminally ill cancer patients in palliative home care. *Palliative and Supportive Care*, 9: 173–80.

Fulford, K.W.M., Dickenson, D.L. and Murray, T.H. (eds) (2002) *Healthcare Ethics and Human Values: an introductory text with readings and case studies.* Oxford: Wiley-Blackwell.

Furedi, F. (1997) *Culture of Fear: risk-taking and the morality of low expectation.* London: Cassell.

Gale, T., Hawley, J. and Sivakumaran, T. (2003) Do mental health professionals really understand probability? Implications for risk assessment and evidence-based practice. *Journal of Mental Health*, 12(4): 417–30.

Gallagher, A. (2013) Values for contemporary nursing practice: waving or drowning? *Nursing Ethics*, 20(6): 615–16.

Gallagher, A. (2012) Slow ethics for nursing practice. *Nursing Ethics*, 19(6): 711–13.

Garrett, T.M., Baillie, H.W. and Garrett, R.M. (2001) *Health Care Ethics: principles and problems*, 4th ed. Englewood Cliffs, NJ:Prentice Hall, Inc.

Gastmans, C. (1999) Care as a moral attitude in nursing. *Nursing Ethics*, 6(3): 214–23.

Gastmans, C., Dierckx de Casterle, B. and Schotsmans, P. (1998) Nursing considered as moral practice: a philosophical-ethical interpretation of nursing. *Kennedy Institute of Ethics Journal*, 8(1): 43–69.

Gert, B., Culver, C.M. and Clouser, K.D. (1997) *Bioethics. A return to the fundamentals.* Oxford: Oxford University Press.

Gilbert, P. (2009) *The Compassionate Mind.* London: Constable.

Gillon, R. (2003) Ethics needs principles – four can encompass the rest – and respect for autonomy should be "first among equals". *Journal of Medical Ethics*, 29: 307–12.

Gillon, R. (1986) *Philosophical Medical Ethics.* Chichester: John Wiley & Sons.

Gilson, L. (2006) Trust in health care: theoretical perspectives and research needs. *Journal of Health Organization and Management*, 20(5): 359–75.

GMC (2009) *Confidentiality.* London: GMC.

GMC (2008) *Consent: patients and doctors making decisions together.* London: GMC.

GMC (2007) *0–18 Years: guidance for all doctors.* London: GMC.

Guilliland, K. and Pairman, S. (1995) *The Midwifery Partnership: a model for practice.* Monograph Series, 95/1 Department of Nursing and Midwifery, Victoria University of Wellington, Wellington, New Zealand.

Handy, C.B. (1997) *Understanding Organizations*, 4th ed. London: Penguin Business.

Harris, J. (1985) *The Value of Life. An introduction to medical ethics.* Routledge: London. Particularly Chapters 10 and 11.

Häyry, M. (2004) Another look at dignity. *Cambridge Quarterly of Healthcare Ethics*, 13: 7–14.

Hayward, J. (1975) *Information – a prescription against pain.* London: Royal College of Nursing. (RCN research series).

Health and Care Professions Council (2017) *Standards of Proficiency for Social Workers in England.* London: HCPC.

Health and Care Professions Council (2016) *Standards of Conduct, Performance and Ethics.* London: HCPC. Available at www.hcpc-uk.org/publications/standards/index.asp?id=38 (accessed 19 January 2017)

Health and Social Care Act 2012, c.7. Available at http://www.legislation.gov.uk/ukpga/2012/7/contents/enacted (accessed 4 January 2017)

Health and Social Care Information Centre (HSCIC) (2013) *A Guide to Confidentiality in Health and Social Care.* Version 1.1. Available at www.digital.nhs.uk/article/1226/A-Guide-to-Confidentiality-in-Health-and-Social-Care- (accessed 30 January 2017)

Healthcare Commission (2007) *Caring for Dignity: a national report on dignity in care for older people while in hospital.* London: Commission for Healthcare Audit and Inspection.

Health Education England, Skills for Care and Skills for Health (2015) *The Care Certificate Standards.* Available at www.skillsforcare.org.uk/Documents/Learning-and-development/Care-Certificate/The-Care-Certificate-Standards.pdf (accessed 27 January 2017)

The Health Foundation (2014) *Seven practical tools to support dignity and compassion in care.* Newsletter, 11 December 2014. Available at health.org.uk/newsletter/seven-practical-tools-support-dignity-and-compassion-care (accessed 27 January 2017)

Health Research Authority (HRA) (2016) *UK policy framework for health and social care research.* Issued for public consultation (now closed). Available at www.hra.nhs.uk/about-the-hra/

consultations-calls/uk-policy-framework-health-social-care-research-consultation-active/ (accessed 27 January 2017)

Hendrick, J. (2004) *Law and Ethics. Foundations in nursing and health care.* Cheltenham: Nelson Thornes.

Herissone-Kelly, P. (2010) Capacity and consent in England and Wales: the Mental Capacity Act under scrutiny. *Cambridge Quarterly of Healthcare Ethics*, 19(3): 344–52.

Herring, J. (2014) *Medical Law and Ethics*, 5th ed. Oxford: Oxford University Press.

HM Government (2010) *The Equality Strategy – Building a Fairer Britain.* London: Government Equality Office. Available at www.gov.uk/government/publications/equality-strategy (accessed 4 January 2017)

HMSO (2014) *Valuing Every Voice, Respecting Every Right: making the case for the Mental Capacity Act. The Government's response to the House of Lords Select Committee Report on the Mental Capacity Act 2005*, Cm 8884. London: The Stationery Office.

HMSO (2014a) *Care Act 2014.* London: The Stationery Office.

HMSO (2010) *Equality Act 2010.* London: The Stationery Office.

HMSO (2001) *The Health and Social Care Act.* London: The Stationery Office.

Hojat, M. (2009) Ten approaches for enhancing empathy in health and human services cultures. *Journal of Health & Human Services Administration*, 31(4): 412–50.

Holland, S. (2010) Scepticism about the virtue ethics approach to nursing ethics. *Nursing Philosophy*, 11: 151–8.

Hollomotz, A. (2014) Are we *Valuing People's* choices *Now*? Restrictions to mundane choices made by adults with learning difficulties. *British Journal of Social Work*, 44: 234–51.

House of Lords Select Committee on the Mental Capacity Act 2005 (2014) *Mental Capacity Act 2005: post-legislative scrutiny*, HL Paper 139, Report of Session 2013–14. London, The Stationery Office.

Human Rights in Healthcare (2012) *The Human Rights in Healthcare Programme 2011–2012.* Liverpool: Mersey Care NHS Trust. Available at www.humanrightsinhealthcare.nhs.uk/About-Us/human_rights_in_healthcarereprot_ld.aspx (accessed 4 January 2014)

Hupcey, J.E. and Miller, J. (2006) Community dwelling adults' perception of interpersonal trust vs. trust in health care providers. *Journal of Clinical Nursing* 15: 1132–9.

Innes, A. (2009) *Dementia Studies. A social science perspective.* London: Sage Publications.

Jackson, A. and Irwin, W. (2011) Dignity, humanity and equality: principle of nursing practice A, *Nursing Standard*, 25(28): 35–7.

Jackson, D., Hickman, L.D., Hutchinson, M. *et al.* (2014) Whistleblowing: an integrative literature review of data-based studies involving nurses. *Contemporary Nurse*, 48(2): 240–52.

Jackson, E. (2013) *Medical Law. Text, cases and materials*, 3rd ed. Oxford: Oxford University Press.

Jacobson, N. (2009) Dignity violation in health care. *Qualitative Health Research*, 19(11): 1536–47.

Jacobson, N. (2007) Dignity and health: a review. *Social Science and Medicine*, 64: 292–302.

Joffe, H. (2003) Risk: from perception to representation. *British Journal of Social Psychology*, 42: 55–73.

Johns, C. and Freshwater, D. (eds) (2005) *Transforming Nursing Through Reflective Practice*, 2nd ed. Oxford: Blackwell.

Johnstone, M.-J. (2009) *Bioethics: a nursing perspective*, 5th ed. Chatswood, New South Wales: Churchill Livingstone Elsevier.

Jones, C. (2003) The utilitarian argument for medical confidentiality: a pilot study of patients' views. *Journal of Medical Ethics*, 29: 348–52.

Karakowsky, L. and Elangovan, A. (2001) Risky decision making in mixed gender teams. Whose tolerance counts? *Small Group Research*, 32(1): 94–111.

Kemshall, H. and Pritchard, J. (eds) (1996) *Good Practice in Risk Assessment and Risk Management, volume 1*. London: Jessica Kingsley.

Kendrick, K.D. and Robinson, S. (2012) 'Tender loving care' as a relational ethic in nursing practice. *Nursing Ethics*, 9(3): 291–300.

Kennedy, H., Shannon, M., Chuahorm U. and Kravetz, M. (2004) The landscape of caring for women: a narrative study of midwifery practice. *Journal of Midwifery and Women's Health*, 49(1): 14–23.

Keogh, B. (2013) *Review into the Quality of Care and Treatment Provided by 14 Hospital Trusts in England: overview report*. Available at www.nhs.uk/NHSEngland/bruce-keogh-review/Documents/outcomes/keogh-review-final-report.pdf (accessed 4 January 2017)

Killmister, S. (2010) Dignity: not such a useless concept. *Journal Medical Ethics*, 36: 160–4.

Kirkham, M. (ed.) (2010) *The Midwife–Mother Relationship*, 2nd ed. Basingstoke: Palgrave Macmillan.

Kitwood, T. (1997) *Dementia Reconsidered: the person comes first*. Milton Keynes: Open University Press.

Kitwood, T. (1993) Person and process in dementia. *International Journal of Psychiatry*, 8: 541–5.

Kolb. D. (1984) *Experiential Learning: experience as the source of learning and development*. London: Prentice-Hall.

Leap, N. (2000) The less we do, the more we give. *In* Kirkham, M. (2000) *The Midwife–Mother Relationship*. Basingstoke: Palgrave Macmillan, Ch.1, pp.17–36.

Levenson, R. (2007) *The Challenge of Dignity in Care: upholding the rights of the individual*. London: Help the Aged.

Lockwood, M. (1985) *Moral Dilemmas in Modern Medicine*. Oxford: Oxford University Press.

Lupton, C. and Croft-White, C. (2013) *Respect and Protect: the experience of older people and staff in care homes and hospitals*. The Panicoa Summary Report. London: Comic Relief. Available at www.nationalcareforum.org.uk/documentLibraryDownload.asp?documentID=1295 (accessed 25 January 2017)

Mackenzie, C. and Rogers, W. (2013) Autonomy, vulnerability and capacity: a philosophical appraisal of the Mental Capacity Act. *International Journal of Law in Context*, 9(1): 37–52.

Mackenzie, C. and Stoljar, N. (eds) (2000) *Relational Autonomy. Feminist perspectives on autonomy, agency and the social self.* New York: Oxford University Press.

Macklin, R. (2003) Dignity is a useless concept: it means no more than respect for persons or their autonomy. *BMJ,* 327(7249): 1419–20.

Matiti, M.R. (2002) *Patient Dignity in Nursing. A phenomenological study.* Unpublished PhD thesis. Huddersfield: University of Huddersfield.

Matiti, M.R. and Baillie, L. (2011) *Dignity in Healthcare: a practical approach for nurses and midwives.* London: Radcliffe.

McLeod, C. (2006) Trust. *In* the *Stanford Encyclopedia of Philosophy.* Available at http://plato.stanford.edu/entries/trust/ (accessed 4 January 2017)

McLeod, C. (2002) *Self-Trust and Reproductive Autonomy.* Cambridge, MA: The MIT Press.

McLeod, C. and Sherwin, S. (2000) 'Relational Autonomy, Self-Trust and Health Care for Patients who are Oppressed' in MacKenzie, C. and Stoljar, N. (eds) *Relational Autonomy. Feminist perspectives on autonomy, agency and the social self.* New York: Oxford University Press.

Mencap (2012) *Death by Indifference: 74 deaths and counting.* A progress report 5 years on. London: Mencap.

Mencap (2007) *Death by Indifference: following up the* Treat me right! *report.* London: Mencap.

Mental Capacity Act (2005) c.9. London: HMSO.

Michael, J. (2008) *Healthcare for All: report of the independent inquiry into access to healthcare for people with learning disabilities.* London: Aldridge Press.

Middleton, J. (2013) Mid Staffs nurse whistleblower made ambassador for cultural change. *Nursing Times.Net.* Available at www.nursingtimes.net/nursing-practice/specialisms/whistleblowing/mid-staffs-nurse-whistleblower-made-ambassador-for-cultural-change/5057408.article (accessed 4 January 2017)

Mill, J.S. (1859) *On Liberty.* London, Longmans Greens and Co.

Morse, J.M., Bottorff, J., Anderson, G., O'Brien, B. and Solberg, S. (2006) Beyond empathy: expanding expressions of caring. *Journal of Advanced Nursing,* 53(1): 75–90.

Morse, J.M., Bottorff, J.L., Anderson, G., O'Brien, B. and Solberg, S. (1992) Beyond empathy: expanding expressions of caring. *Journal of Advanced Nursing,* 17: 809–21.

National Dignity Council (2015) *The Dignity in Care Campaign.* Birmingham: National Dignity Council. Available at www.dignityincare.org.uk/About/Dignity_in_Care_campaign/ (accessed 4 January 2017)

National Voices (2014) *Person centred care 2020. Calls and contributions from health and social care charities.* London: National Voices. Available at www.nationalvoices.org.uk/sites/default/files/public/publications/person-centred-care-2020.pdf (accessed 27 January 2017)

Niemeijer, A., Depla, M., Frederiks, B. and Hertog, C. (2015) The experiences of people with dementia and intellectual disabilities with surveillance technologies in residential care. *Nursing Ethics,* 22(3): 307–20.

NHS (2014) *Five Year Forward View.* Available at www.england.nhs.uk/wp-content/uploads/2014/10/5yfv-web.pdf (accessed 17 February 2017)

NHS Leadership Academy (2013) *Nine Dimensions of Leadership.* Leeds: NHS Leadership Academy.

NHS Publications (2016) *Leading Change, Adding Value: a framework for nursing, midwifery and care staff.* Available at www.england.nhs.uk/wp-content/uploads/2016/05/nursing-framework.pdf (accessed 2 December 2016)

Nordenfelt, L. (2003b) Dignity and the Care of the Elderly. *Medicine, Health Care and Philosophy*, 6, 2, pp.103–110.

NMC (2015) *The Code: professional standards of practice and behaviour for nurses and midwives.* London: NMC. Available at www.nmc-uk.org/Documents/NMC-Publications/revised-new-NMC-Code.pdf (accessed 4 January 2017)

NMC (2014) *The Code: standards of conduct, performance and ethics for nurses and midwives. Draft revised version* for consultation. London: NMC. Available at www.nmc-uk.org/Get-involved/Consultations/Consultation-on-revalidation-and-the-revised-Code/ (accessed 4 January 2017)

NMC (2010a) *Standards for pre-registration nursing education.* London: NMC. Available at www.nmc.org.uk/globalassets/sitedocuments/standards/nmc-standards-for-pre-registration-nursing-education.pdf (accessed 4 January 2017)

NMC (2010b) *Standards for competence for registered nurses.* London: NMC. Available at www.nmc-uk.org/Publications/Standards/ (accessed 4 January 2017)

NMC (2008) *The Code: Standards of conduct, performance and ethics for nurses and midwives.* London: NMC. Available at www.nmc-uk.org/Documents/Standards/The-code-A4-20100406.pdf (accessed 4 January 2017)

Nolan, M., Ryan, T., Enderby, P. and Reid, D. (2002) Towards a more inclusive vision of dementia care practice and research. *Dementia: The International Journal of Social Research and Practice*, 1: 193–211.

Nordenfelt, L. (2004) The varieties of dignity. *Health Care Analysis*, 12: 69–81.

Nouwen, H.J., McNeil, D.P. and Morrison, D.A. (1982) *Compassion: a reflection on the Christian life.* London: Darton, Longman and Todd.

Nuffield Council on Bioethics (2009) *Dementia: ethical issues.* London: Nuffield Council on Bioethics.

Nussbaum, M. (2001) *Upheavals of Thought: the intelligence of emotions.* New York: Cambridge University Press.

Nussbaum, M. (1996) Compassion: the basic social emotion. *Social Philosophy and Policy Foundation*, 13(1): 27–58.

Oelofsen, N. (2012) *Developing Reflective Practice.* Banbury: Lantern Publishing.

O'Neill, O. (2002) *A Question of Trust. The BBC Reith Lectures 2002* Cambridge: Cambridge University Press. Available as transcripts at www.bbc.co.uk/radio4/reith2002/lectures.shtml (accessed 4 January 2017)

O'Neill, O. (2002a) A Question of Trust. Spreading Suspicion. *Reith Lectures 2002* Lecture 1. BBC Radio 4 transcript available at www.bbc.co.uk/radio4/reith2002/lectures.shtml (accessed 4 January 2017)

O'Neill, O. (2002b) A Question of Trust. Trust and Terror. *Reith Lectures 2002* Lecture 2. BBC Radio 4 transcript available at www.bbc.co.uk/radio4/reith2002/lectures.shtml (accessed 4 January 2017)

O'Neill, O. (2002c) A Question of Trust. Trust and Transparency. *Reith Lectures 2002* Lecture 4. BBC Radio 4 transcript available at www.bbc.co.uk/radio4/reith2002/lectures.shtml (accessed 4 January 2017)

Owens, J. and Cribb, A. (2013) Beyond choice and individualism: understanding autonomy for public health ethics. *Public Health Ethics*, 6(3): 262–71.

Oxford English Dictionary (2nd ed) (1989) Simpson, J.A. and Weiner, E.S.C. (eds). Oxford: Clarendon Press.

Page, L. (2003) One-to-one midwifery: restoring the "with woman" relationship in midwifery. *Journal of Midwifery and Women's Health*, 48(2): 119–25.

Parliamentary and Health Service Ombudsman (PHSO) (2011) *Care and compassion? Report of the Health Service Ombudsman on ten investigations into NHS care of older people*, HC 778. London: The Stationery Office.

Pattison, S. (2004) Understanding values. *In* Pattison, S. and Pill, R. (eds) (2004) *Values in Professional Practice. Lessons for health, social care and other professionals.* Oxford: Radcliffe Medical Press.

Pellegrino, E.D. and Thomasma, D.C. (1988) *For the Patient's Good: the restoration of beneficence in health care.* New York: Oxford University Press.

Pergert, P. and Lützén, K. (2012) Balancing truth-telling in the preservation of hope: a relational ethics approach. *Nursing Ethics*, 19(1): 21–9.

Peters, M.A. (2006) Compassion: an investigation into the experience of nursing faculty. *International Journal for Human Caring*, 10(3): 38–46.

Pidgeon, N., Hood, C., Turner, B. and Gibson, R. (1992) Risk perception. *In* The Royal Society's *Risk: analysis, perception and management – report of a Royal Society Study Group.* London: The Royal Society.

Policy Research Institute on Ageing & Ethnicity (PRIAE) (2001) *Towards Dignity: acting on the lessons from black and minority ethnic older people's experiences of hospital care. A Report from PRIAE for the Help the Aged Dignity on the Ward Campaign.* London: Help the Aged. Available at www.priae.org/assets/palcope/PRIAE_Hospital_Care_Dignity_on_the_Ward_Help_the_Aged_2001.pdf (accessed 4 January 2017)

Pols, J. (2013) Washing the patient: dignity and aesthetic values in nursing care. *Nursing Philosophy*, 14(3): 186–200.

Prideaux, A. (2011) Issues in nursing documentation and record-keeping practice. *British Journal of Nursing*, 20(22): 1450.

Quallington, J. (2011) *What is Good Care? Service users' and carers' interpretation.* Unpublished report. IMPACT Service User and Carer Group, University of Worcester.

RCN (2013) *Dignity in Health Care for People with Learning Disabilities*, 2nd ed. RCN guidance. London: RCN.

RCN (2012) *Health Inequalities and the Social Determinants of Health*. Policy Briefing 01/12. Available at www2.rcn.org.uk/__data/assets/pdf_file/0007/438838/01.12_Health_inequalities_and_the_social_determinants_of_health.pdf (accessed 27 January 2017)

RCN (2011) *Principles of Care. The principles of nursing practice*. London: RCN Publishing Company.

RCN (2011a) *Principles of Care. Principle A: dignity, humanity and equality*. London: RCN Publishing Company (see Jackson, A. and Irwin, W. (2011) Dignity, humanity and equality: principle of Nursing Practice A. *Nursing Standard*, 25(28): 35–7).

RCN (2008) *Defending Dignity – challenges and opportunities for nursing*. Available at www.rcn.org.uk/__data/assets/pdf_file/0011/166655/003257.pdf (accessed 4 January 2017)

Rethink Mental Illness (2017) *NHS Treatment – Your Rights*. Available at www.rethink.org/living-with-mental-illness/rights-restrictions/nhs-treatment-your-rights/rights (accessed 17 February 2017)

Rolfe, G. (2001) *Critical Reflection for Nursing and the HELPING Professions: a user's guide*. Basingstoke: Palgrave.

Schantz, M.L. (2007) Compassion: a concept analysis. *Nursing Forum*, 42(2): 48–55.

Schermer, M. (2007) Nothing but the truth? On truth and deception in dementia care. *Bioethics*, 21(1): 13–22.

Schön, D. (1987) *Educating the Reflective Practitioner*. London: Jossey Bass.

Schroeder, D. (2010) Dignity: one, two, three, four, five, still counting. *Cambridge Quarterly of Healthcare Ethics*, 19: 118–25.

Schulz, R., Hebert, R.S., Dew, M.A. *et al.* (2007) Patient suffering and caregiver compassion: new opportunities for research, practice, and policy. *Gerontologist*, 47(1): 4–13.

Seedhouse, D. (2009) *Ethics: the heart of health care*, 3rd ed. Chichester: John Wiley & Sons.

Seedhouse, D. (1998) *Ethics: the heart of health care*, 2nd ed. Chichester: John Wiley & Sons.

Seedhouse, D. and Gallagher, A. (2002) Undignifying institutions. *Journal of Medical Ethics*, 28: 368–72.

Sellman, D. (2011) *What makes a good nurse. Why the virtues are important for nurses*. London: Jessica Kingsley.

Sellman, D. (2006) The importance of being trustworthy. *Nursing Ethics*, 13(2): 105–15.

Sherwin, S. (1998) A relational approach to autonomy in health care. *In* The Feminist Health Care Ethics Research Network, coordinator Sherwin, S. (ed.) *The Politics of Women's Health: exploring agency and autonomy*. Philadelphia: Temple University Press.

Siddiqui, J. (1999) The therapeutic relationship in midwifery. *British Journal of Midwifery*, 7: 111–14.

Simons, L., Tee, S. and Coldham, T. (2010) Developing values-based education through service user participation. *The Journal of Mental Health Training, Education and Practice*, 5(1): 20–7.

Singer, P. (1993) *Practical Ethics*, 2nd ed. Cambridge: Cambridge University Press.

Skills for Care (2014) *Adult social care workforce recruitment and retention strategy*, 2nd ed. Leeds: Skills for Care. Available at www.skillsforcare.org.uk (accessed 4 January 2017)

Skills for Care (2013) *Common core principles to support dignity in adult social care.* Leeds: Skills for Care. Available at www.skillsforcare.org.uk/Skills/Dignity/Dignity.aspx (accessed 4 January 2017)

Skills for Care and Skills for Health (2013a) *Code of Conduct for Healthcare Support Workers and Adult Social Care Workers in England.* Leeds and Bristol: Skills for Care and Skills for Health. Available at www.skillsforcare.org.uk/Document-library/Standards/National-minimum-training-standard-and-code/CodeofConduct.pdf (accessed 4 January 2017)

Skills for Care and Skills for Health (2013b) *Core Competences for Healthcare Support Workers and Adult Social Care Workers in England.* Leeds and Bristol: Skills for Care and Skills for Health.

Smith, C. (2005) Understanding trust and confidence: two paradigms and their significance for health and social care. *Journal of Applied Philosophy*, 22(3): 299–316.

Snelling, P. (2014) What's wrong with tombstoning and what does this tell us about responsibility for health? *Public Health Ethics*, 2: 144–57.

Snow, N.E. (1991) Compassion. *American Philosophical Quarterly*, 28(3): 195–205.

Social Care Institute for Excellence (SCIE) (2013) Dignity factors. In the updated *Practice Guide for Adult Services Guide 15: Dignity in care.* London: SCIE. Available at www.scie.org.uk/publications/guides/guide15/factors/index.asp (accessed 4 January 2017)

Social Care Institute for Excellence (SCIE) (2006) *Practice Guide for Adult Services Guide 09: Dignity in care.* London: SCIE.

Straughair, C. (2012a) Exploring compassion: implications for contemporary nursing. Part 1. *British Journal of Nursing*, 21(3): 160–4.

Straughair, C. (2012b) Exploring compassion: implications for contemporary nursing. Part 2. *British Journal of Nursing*, 21(4): 239–44.

Tadd, W. (2005) Dignity and older Europeans. *Quality in ageing: policy, practice and research*, 6(1): 2–5.

Tadd, W. (2004) *Dignity and Older Europeans: comparative analysis of data from older people's focus groups from all centres.* Deliverable 9. Cardiff: University of Cardiff. Available at www.cardiff.ac.uk/socsi/dignity/europe/older_peoples_views.pdf (accessed 4 January 2017)

Tadd, W., Hillman, A., Calnan, S., *et al.* (2011) *Dignity in Practice: an exploration of the care of older adults in acute NHS Trusts.* NIHR Service Delivery and Organisation Programme. Project 08/1819/218. NETSCC. Southampton: SDO. Available at https://njl-admin.nihr.ac.uk/document/download/2008912 (accessed 27 January 2017)

Tadd, W., Hillman, A., Calnan, S., *et al.* (2011a) *Dignity in Practice: an exploration of the care of older adults in acute NHS Trusts. (A research summary).* NIHR Service Delivery and Organisation Programme. Available at www.cardiff.ac.uk/socsi/dignity/dignityinpractice/cesagen-dip-research-summary.pdf (accessed 4 January 2017)

Tadd, W., Vanlaere, L. and Gastmans, C. (2010) Clarifying the concept of human dignity in the care of the elderly: a dialogue between empirical and philosophical approaches. *Ethical Perspectives*, 17(1): 253–81.

Tadd, W., Bayer, T. and Dieppe, P. (2002) Dignity in health care: reality or rhetoric. *Reviews in Clinical Gerontology*, 12(1): 1–4.

Tambuyzer, E. and van Audenhove, C. (2015) Is perceived patient involvement in mental health care associated with satisfaction and empowerment? *Health Expectations*, 18(4): 516–26.

Taylor, H. (2013) Determining capacity to consent to treatment. *Nursing Times*, 109(43): 12–14.

Thom, D.H. and Campbell, B. (1997) Patient–physician trust: an exploratory study. *Journal of Family Practice*, 44: 169–76.

Thompson, N. (2011) *Promoting Equality: working with diversity and difference.* Basingstoke: Palgrave Macmillan.

Thompson, N. (2006) *Anti-discriminatory Practice*, 4th ed. Basingstoke: Palgrave.

Tilmouth, T. and Quallington, J. (2016) *Level 5 Diploma in Leadership for Health and Social Care*, 2nd ed. London: Hodder Education.

Tingle, J. and Cribb, A. (eds) (2013) *Nursing Law and Ethics*, 4th ed. London: Wiley-Blackwell.

Titterton, M. (2005) *Risk and Risk Taking in Health and Social Welfare.* London: Jessica Kingsley Publishing.

Tong, R. (1998) The ethics of care: a feminist virtue ethics of care for health practitioners. *Journal of Medicine and Philosophy*, 23(2): 131–52.

Toon, P.D. (1999) The cultivation of virtue. *Royal College of General Practitioners Occasional Paper*, Ch. 9, 78: 57–63.

Trevithick, P. (2005) *Social Work Skills: a practice handbook*, 2nd ed. Buckinghamshire, Open University Press.

Tschudin, V. (2003) *Ethics in Nursing. The caring relationship*, 3rd ed. Edinburgh: Butterworth Heinemann.

Tuckett, A. (2004) Truth-telling in clinical practice and the arguments for and against: a review of the literature. *Nursing Ethics*, 11(5): 500–13.

Twelvetrees, A. (2002) *Community Work*, 3rd ed. Basingstoke: Palgrave.

Uslaner, E. (2001) *Trust as a Moral Value.* Paper presented at the Conference, "Social Capital: Interdisciplinary Perspectives" University of Exeter, 15–20 September.

van der Cingel, M. (2014) Compassion: the missing link in quality of care. *Nurse Education Today*, 34(9): 1253–7.

van der Cingel, M. (2011) Compassion in care: a qualitative study of older people with a chronic disease and nurses. *Nursing Ethics*, 18(5): 672–85.

van der Cingel, M. (2009) Compassion and professional care: exploring the domain. *Nursing Philosophy*, 10(2): 124–36.

von Dietze, E. and Orb, A. (2000) Compassionate care: a moral dimension of nursing. *Nursing Inquiry*, 7: 166–74.

Wainwright, P. and Pattison, S. (2004) What can we expect of professional codes of conduct, practice and ethics? *In* Pattison, S. and Pill, R. (eds) *Values in Professional Practice*. Abingdon: Radcliffe Publishing.

Walton, A.M. and Alvarez, M. (2010) Imagine: compassion fatigue training for nurses. *Clinical Journal of Oncology Nursing*, 14(4): 399–400.

Warburton, N. (2001) *Freedom. An introduction with readings*. London: Routledge.

Warren, M. (1973) On the legal and moral status of abortion. *The Monist*, 57: 43–61.(Revised version in LaFollette, H. (ed) (1997) *Ethics in Practice. An anthology*. Oxford: Blackwell Publishers.

Watson, J. (2012) *Human Caring Science: a theory of nursing*, 2nd ed. Sudbury, MA: Jones & Bartlett Learning.

Welie, J.V.M. and Welie, S.P.K. (2001) Patient Decision Making Competence: outlines of a conceptual analysis. *Medicine, Health Care and Philosophy*, 4(2): 127–38.

West, M., Dawson, J. and Kaur, M. (2015) *Making the Difference: diversity and inclusion in the NHS*. London: King's Fund. Available at www.kingsfund.org.uk/sites/files/kf/field/field_publication_file/Making-the-difference-summary-Kings-Fund-Dec-2015.pdf (accessed 17 February 2017)

West, M., Eckert, R., Steward, K. and Pasmore, B. (2014) *Developing Collective Leadership for Health Care*. London: King's Fund.

Whitehead, J. and Wheeler, H. (2008) Patients' experience of privacy and dignity. Part 2: an empirical study. *British Journal of Nursing*, 17(7): 458–64.

Willis Commission (2012) *Quality with Compassion: The Future of Nursing Education. Report of the Willis Commission*. London: Royal College of Nursing.

Wilson, F., Ingleton, C., Gott, M. and Gardiner, C. (2014) Autonomy and choice in palliative care: time for a new model? *Journal of Advanced Nursing*, 70(5): 1020–9.

Woodbridge, K. and Fulford, K.W. (2004) *Whose Values? A workbook for values-based practice in mental health care*. London: The Sainsbury Centre for Mental Health.

Woolhead, G., Calnan, M., Dieppe, P. and Tadd, W. (2004) Dignity in older age: what do older people in the United Kingdom think? *Age and Ageing*, 33(2): 165–70.

Youngson, R. (2014) Re-inspiring compassionate caring: the reawakening purpose workshop. *Journal of Compassionate Health Care*. Available open access via BioMed Central at www.jcompassionatehc.com/content/1/1/1 (accessed 5 January 2017)

Youngson, R. (2012) *Time to Care. How to love your patients and your job*. New Zealand: Rebelheart Publishers.

Youngson, R. (2008) *Compassion in Healthcare: the missing dimension of healthcare reform?* Futures Debate, May 2008, Paper 2. London: NHS Confederation. Available at www.nhsconfed.org/~/media/Confederation/Files/Publications/Documents/Compassion%20in%20healthcare.pdf (accessed 5 January 2017)

INDEX